S.T.D.

Sexually Transmitted Diseases

including HIV/AIDS

by

John T. Daugirdas, MD

Third edition.   Copyright © 1992 by John T. Daugirdas
Published by Medtext, Inc.,
15W560 89th St.
Hinsdale, Illinois, USA 60521   tel: (708) 325-3277

***

Library of Congress Catalog Card Number 92-090770
Printed in the United States of America

Second Printing, 1993

Daugirdas, John T., 1949-
  STD: sexually transmitted diseases, including HIV/AIDS/ by John T. Daugirdas, MD. -
p. cm.
  ISBN 0-9629279-1-0

  1. Sexually transmitted diseases -- Juvenile literature. I.
Title.

RC200.2   616.951   --
                                                         MARC

The paper used in this publication meets the minimum requirements of the American National Standard for Information Sciences -- Permanence of Paper for Printed Library Materials, ANSI Z39.48-1984.
***

Warning -- Disclaimer:
This book is designed to provide information in regard to the subject matter covered. It is sold with the understanding that the publisher, authors, and advisors are not rendering medical or professional services. Medicine is a rapidly changing area. All efforts have been made to provide information that is medically correct at the time of publication. However, there may be mistakes, both typographical and in content. For this reason, this text should be used only as a general guide and not as the ultimate source of information. All questions concerning diagnosis, treatment, and partner notification of STDs, as well as prevention, should be discussed with your doctor or clinic. The authors, advisors, and publisher shall have neither liability nor responsibility to any person or entity with respect to any loss or damage caused or alleged to be caused directly or indirectly by the information contained in this book.

Preface

"Sexually Transmitted Diseases" by Dr. John Daugirdas provides the reader with an easy-to-understand overview of common sexually transmitted illnesses. The book outlines basic information about these infections including methods of transmission, common symptoms, treatment, and long-term complications in a frank and easy-to-understand style. The illustrations are clear and complement the text.

Many sexually transmitted diseases continue to increase at an alarming rate. Education concerning the prevention of these infections is vital. This text is an important addition to that effort.

Larry J. Goodman, M.D.
Associate Professor of Medicine
Section of Infectious Diseases
Rush-Presbyterian St. Luke's Medical Center
Chicago, IL

Introduction

The first edition of this book, prepared in 1977, was an attempt by me as a physician just out of medical school to educate young men and women about sexually transmitted diseases. I was attending at several emergency rooms at the time, and was shocked by the number of patients with preventable pelvic inflammatory disease that were seeking medical attention. Without exception, the young patients I was treating were dangerously uninformed about sexually transmitted infections. Much of the educational material available then was either too complex to be easily understandable, or too superficial to be useful. I thought perhaps I could do better. The material was simplified to focus on the principal STDs, and prevention and partner notification were emphasized. Sections giving specific recommendations regarding type of physician to see, what to expect at the doctor's office, etc., were included. All forms of sexual behavior leading to risk were discussed. To help hold interest in a subject that is inherently repelling and frightening, the wry humor of Montreal-based graphic designer Pierre Durand was enlisted.

The second edition, printed in 1991, was a complete rewrite. It incorporated new information about HIV and genital warts. The second edition was prepared with the gracious help of Ms. Beverly Biehr and the staff and advisors of the Bureau of Science of the Chicago Public Schools.

The third edition represents an incremental improvement. The reading level was lowered. Several of the graphics and cartoons were modified to enhance clarity as well as acceptability. Photos of STD lesions were added. The suggestions of Dr. Mary Spink Neumann at the Centers for Disease Control (Atlanta, Georgia, USA) and those of many other health educators are gratefully acknowledged.

John T. Daugirdas, M.D., F.A.C.P

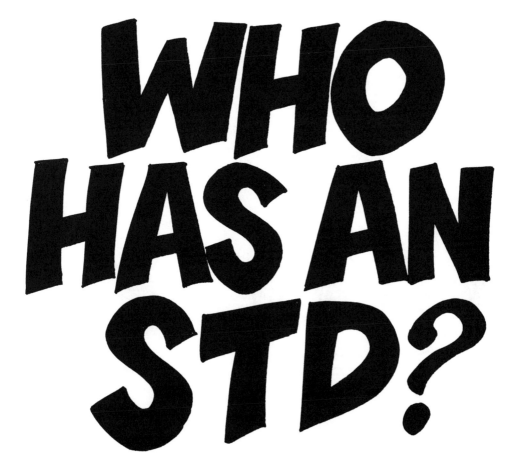

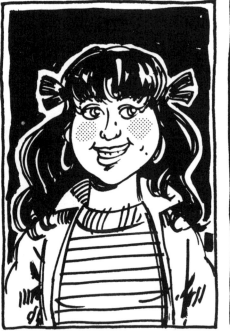

Rosita?

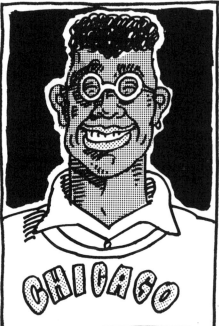

Bobby Jones?

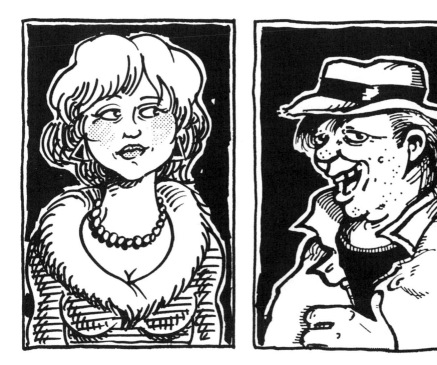

Mary Jane?   Sammy?

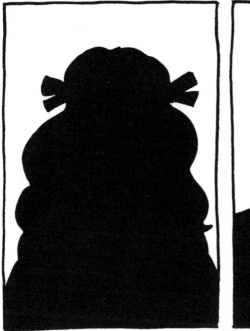

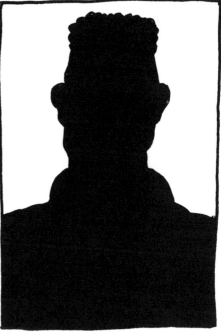

Yes!
Rosita:
Fourteen years old, and
having sex only with her
one true love.

Yes!
Robert T. Jones:
An "all - A" student
who has many fans.

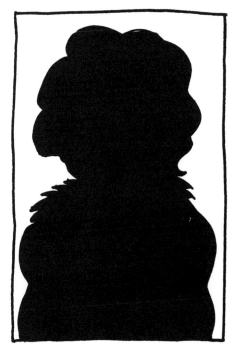
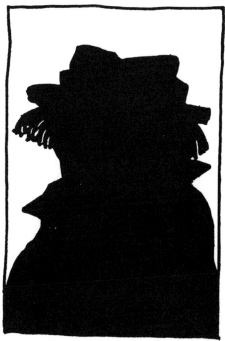

Yes!
Mary Jane:
On a fast-track career.
She got an STD after going
a bit too far at one of those
wild office parties.

NO!
Sammy:
He has a lot of free time.
He doesn't do drugs, though.
He hasn't had intimate
sexual contact in years!

Who has an STD?

Any person, from any social class or race, no matter how old they are, can get one of these infections. How? By having intimate sexual contact with an infected partner. Some STDs you can get by abuse of injectable drugs, if you share a needle or syringe with an infected partner.

This book will tell you what an STD is. It will describe how STDs can be spread. You will find out how your doctor or clinic can test for an STD. You will read about how STDs can be treated. You will find out how to avoid actions that put you at risk for getting an STD.

Table of Contents

Part one   **Basic information**

What is an STD?   1

Signs and symptoms
  Chlamydia and gonorrhea   13
  Syphilis   20
  Herpes-2   22
  Genital warts (HPV)   25
  HIV and AIDS   27
Review   32

Non-STD causes of STD symptoms   37
  Discharge and/or burning   37
  Pain in the lower abdomen   41
  Sores/blisters/pimples/warts   42

During pregnancy   43

Lab tests   47
  Looking under the microscope   49
  Swab tests (cultures)   50
  Checking the blood   52

Treatment   57
  Tests   57
  Antibiotics   57
  Partner notification   58
  What kind of doctor to see   69
  At the doctor's office   71

Part two   **Prevention**
                Abstinence 77
                Mutual monogamy 78
                Danger of using drugs 80
                Latex condoms 83
                Decision making 91
                How to say "NO!" when you don't want to 99

Part three   **Case reports**
                Spring Break 103
                Party 105
                Macho Man 107
                Time Bomb 109

Part four   **Appendices**
                1. Other causes of burning and increased
                    discharge in the vaginal area 113
                      Cystitis 113
                      Candida (yeast) 114
                      Trichomonas 115
                      Gardnerella 116
                2. Other causes of pimples, blisters,
                    and sores on the genitals 119
                3. Scabies 125
                4. Pubic lice (pediculosis) 127
                5. Viral hepatitis 129

Glossary 133

Review questions 137

AIDS Hotlines for English-speaking countries 147

Part one

Basic information

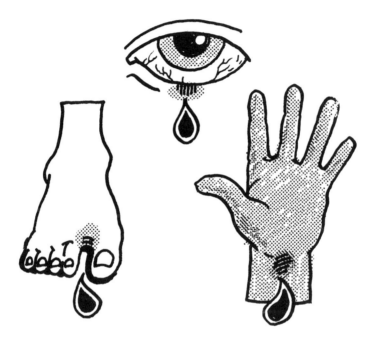

What is an STD?

S.T.D. stands for **S**exually **T**ransmitted **D**isease. STDs used to be called *venereal* diseases. They were named after Venus, the ancient Roman goddess of love. There is nothing lovely about them.

STDs are infections
Infections can appear in any part of the human body. They all are caused by **microbes** that live and grow in the tissues involved. Take a drop of tissue fluid from an infected eye, foot, or hand. Put the drop under a microscope. Often you will see the microbes that are causing the problem.

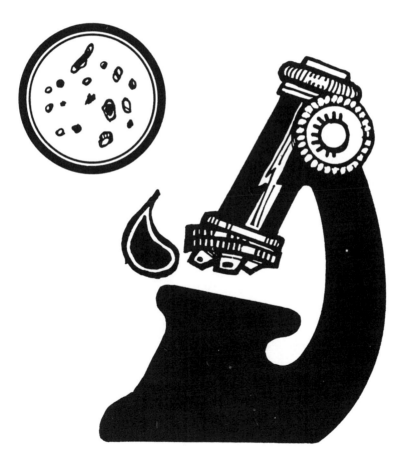

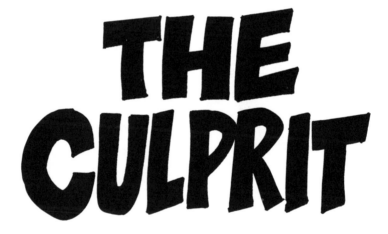

THE
CULPRIT

2

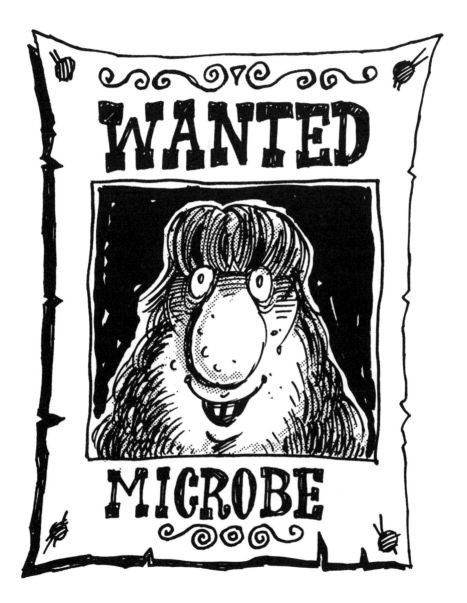

3

Bacteria and viruses

Most STD microbes are bacteria or viruses. A **bacterium** is a microbe that exists as a single cell (or a part of a single cell). A **virus** is a microbe that is made up of molecules that contain DNA or RNA. After it enters a cell, a virus fools the cell. The cell sees the viral DNA or RNA as its own and copies it. In this way the virus can survive, divide, and spread.

Three STDs caused by **bacteria** are Chlamydia, gonorrhea, and syphilis.

STD	Name of Bacteria
CHLAMYDIA	*Chlamydia trachomatis*
GONORRHEA	*Neisseria gonorrhoeae*
SYPHILIS	*Treponema pallidum*

Three STDs caused by **viruses** are herpes-2, genital warts, and <u>A</u>cquired <u>I</u>mmuno-<u>D</u>eficiency <u>S</u>yndrome (AIDS).

STD	Name of Virus
HERPES-2	*Herpes simplex type 2*
GENITAL WARTS	*Human Papilloma Virus (HPV)*
AIDS	*Human Immunodeficiency Virus (HIV)*

These are the six STDs that we will be discussing in the body of this book. Other STDs, including hepatitis, are described in the Appendices.

4

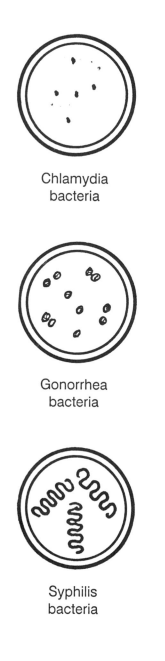

Chlamydia
bacteria

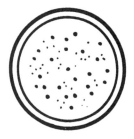

Herpes-2
Virus

Gonorrhea
bacteria

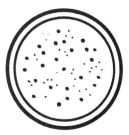

Human Papilloma
Virus

Syphilis
bacteria

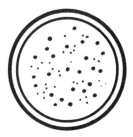

Human Immunodeficiency
Virus

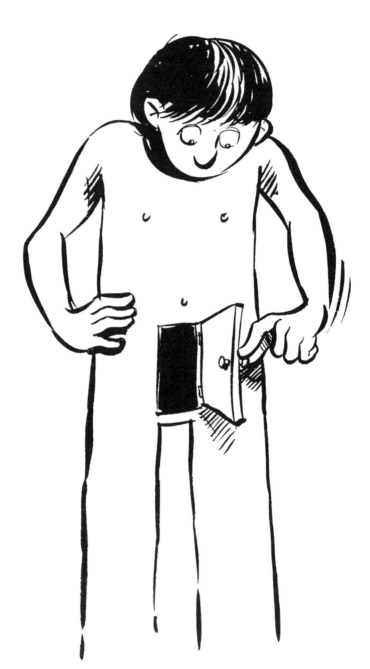

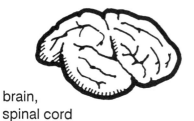

brain,
spinal cord

The danger

STDs cause trouble when they spread out from the genital area. STDs use the genitals as a *doorway* into the body. Once inside, the microbes can cause damage to major body organs.

Women who have an STD while pregnant pose a special problem. Sometimes STD microbes can move into the fetus or spread to the baby during birth.

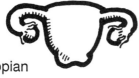

Fallopian
tubes

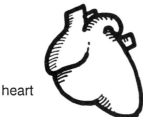

heart

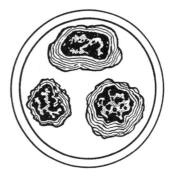

immune
system

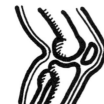

joints

7

How can you get an STD?

There are TWO risk behaviors:

> 1. **Intimate sexual contact**
> 2. **Abuse of injectable drugs**

1. INTIMATE SEXUAL CONTACT = HIGH RISK
Intimate sexual contact is when one person's sex organs (penis or vagina), or anus, touch or enter the openings of another person's body. You can get an STD during **intimate sexual contact** with an infected partner.

Vaginal or anal sex (sexual intercourse) = **HIGH** risk
Vaginal or anal sex occurs when the penis touches or enters the vagina or anus. STD microbes can spread from an infected partner to you during direct touching between the penis and vagina or anus. STD microbes may be present in your partner's semen or vaginal or anal fluid. During vaginal or anal sex, small amounts of genital fluids are exchanged. STD microbes in these fluids can hitch along for the ride and enter your body. Some STDs cause genital or anal sores. STD microbes are present in these sores. The microbes can move into your body when your sex organs come into close contact with the sores.

Oral sex = **MEDIUM** risk
It is not common to get an STD from oral sex, but this can happen. Suppose you perform oral sex (oral sex = touching the partner's penis, vagina, or anus with the mouth, lips, or tongue) on a person with an STD. Semen, or vaginal or anal fluid that may contain STD microbes can enter your mouth. STD microbes can get into your body in this way. Suppose that, with your lips, tongue or mouth, you touch a sore caused by an STD. Some of the STD microbes from the sore can move into your mouth and into your body.

8

Mouth to genital spread of STDs is not common, but it is possible. Some STD microbes can be present in the mouth area. If a person with an STD performs oral sex on you, then STD microbes can spread from his or her mouth to your sex organs and into your body.

<u>Fondling the genitals</u> = **SOME** risk

This is NOT a likely way of getting an STD. However, there can be tiny cuts on the fingers (for instance, at the base of the nail). If your partner has an STD, then the microbes may be present in body fluids in his or her sex organs or rectum. It is possible that these microbes could enter your body through small cuts or bruises on your hands or fingers.

2. ABUSE OF INJECTABLE DRUGS = HIGH risk

Some STD microbes are present in the blood of infected persons. Suppose you inject yourself with drugs or steroids. Suppose you use an unsterilized needle, syringe, or liquid that has been used before you by a person with HIV. These things might have live virus in them. When you use them, you might inject yourself with HIV!

LOW OR NO RISK

<u>Kissing</u> = very low or NO risk

Can **kissing** transmit an STD? The risk is very low as long as no sores are present in the mouth area, BUT:

> See comments about kissing when syphilis sores or herpes-2 sores are present in the mouth area (pages 20 and 22). See comments about kissing and the spread of HIV (page 30).

Holding hands, hugging, touching = NO risk

STD microbes don't infect the skin covering the rest of the body. There is no danger of getting an STD from holding hands, hugging, or touching.

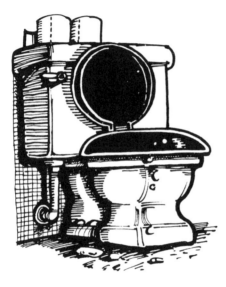

A poor alibi
By the way, STDs are not spread by toilet seats.

Also, you cannot get an STD from towels, doorknobs, or from swimming pools.

Statistics (number of people infected)

<u>What do the numbers show?</u>

CHLAMYDIA	The rate is rising.
GONORRHEA	The rate fell somewhat in the recent past. Now the rate is still high and it is no longer falling.
SYPHILIS	The rate is the highest it's been since 1940. There is a rising number of babies being born with syphilis.
HERPES-2	The rate is rising.
GENITAL WARTS (HPV)	The rate is rising quickly.
AIDS (HIV)	The rate is rising, mostly in young women and in babies.

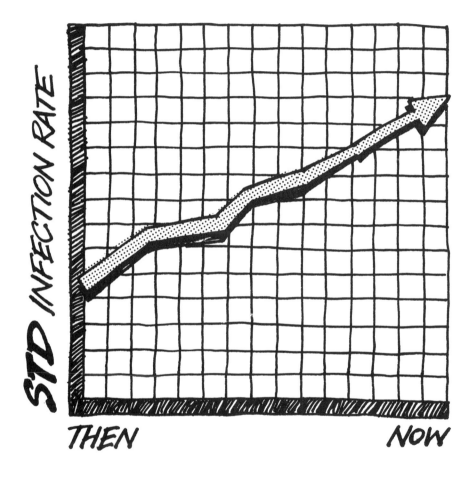

Signs and Symptoms

Before you get really scared...
This section describes symptoms caused by STD microbes. **Other health problems can cause the same type of symptoms!** *Some of these other problems are described in pages 37-42 and in the APPENDIX sections. If you think you have one of the symptoms described here, then go to your doctor or health clinic without delay. There you can find out if your symptoms are due to an STD or if you have some other problem.*

CHLAMYDIA AND GONORRHEA

Infection by Chlamydia or gonorrhea microbes is very common. You can become infected with Chlamydia only. You can get gonorrhea only. You can get both at the same time.

The symptoms caused by these two STDs are pretty much the same. They are described on the pages that follow. Symptoms may be mild or there may be no symptoms. Because of this, persons with Chlamydia or gonorrhea may not know that they have an STD.

Chlamydia and gonorrhea infect the sex organs. They infect the rectum, also. They infect and damage the Fallopian tubes. Gonorrhea microbes also can infect the throat. Once inside the body, they can spread by way of the blood to the joints, skin, and major body organs.

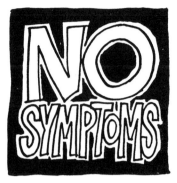

No symptoms

The bad news is that you can have Chlamydia or gonorrhea but have no symptoms at all! Up to 20% of men will have no symptoms.

Up to 80% of women will not have symptoms. In women these microbes like to infect the **cervix** (the neck of the uterus). There are not many nerve fibers in the cervix. For this reason the cervix is not painful when infected. Even a direct look at the cervix by a doctor will not always show that these microbes are present. Special tests (described later) need to be performed.

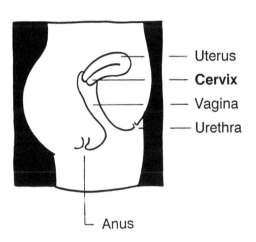

— Uterus

— **Cervix**

— Vagina

— Urethra

Anus

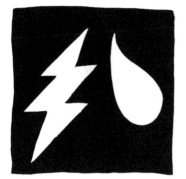

Discharge, burning

More than 80% of the time, men with Chlamydia or gonorrhea do have symptoms. Pus forms at the end of the penis. There is a burning feeling while passing urine. Common names for Chlamydia or gonorrhea include "morning drop" and "the drip". Other names are "the dose", "the clap", and "GC".

Some infected women will have the same kind of symptoms. The normal amount of vaginal discharge is increased (discharge = liquid composed of secretions and/or pus). Also, there is a burning feeling while passing urine. Painful passage of urine occurs when STD microbes infect the **urethra**. The urethra is the tube through which the urine leaves the body.

In the picture above, the drop stands for pus or increased vaginal discharge. The lightning bolt stands for the burning pain that is felt when passing urine.

Women who get increased vaginal discharge or burning when passing urine often DO NOT HAVE AN STD!! Most of the time, the cause is some other health problem (see page 40 and Appendix 1).

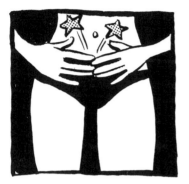

Lower abdominal pain

Women with Chlamydia or gonorrhea sometimes feel pain in the lower abdomen (the part covered by a bikini). Often the pain is first noticed after the end of a menstrual period

Pain here can mean that the microbes have moved up into the Fallopian tubes. The microbes can move up even higher and infect the region around the liver. Then pain also can be felt under the rib cage.

STD infection of the Fallopian tubes does not always cause pain. Sometimes there is no pain and no symptoms of any kind.

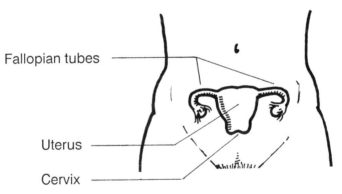

Fallopian tubes

Uterus

Cervix

16

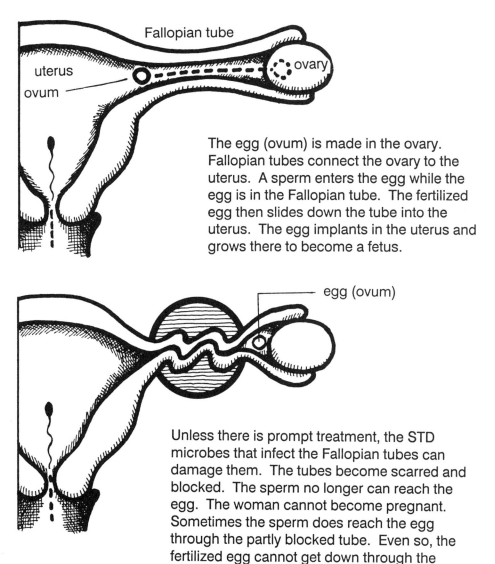

Fallopian tube

uterus

ovum

ovary

The egg (ovum) is made in the ovary. Fallopian tubes connect the ovary to the uterus. A sperm enters the egg while the egg is in the Fallopian tube. The fertilized egg then slides down the tube into the uterus. The egg implants in the uterus and grows there to become a fetus.

egg (ovum)

Unless there is prompt treatment, the STD microbes that infect the Fallopian tubes can damage them. The tubes become scarred and blocked. The sperm no longer can reach the egg. The woman cannot become pregnant. Sometimes the sperm does reach the egg through the partly blocked tube. Even so, the fertilized egg cannot get down through the damaged tube into the uterus. The egg may then try to grow in the Fallopian tube. This is called **ectopic pregnancy**. The growing embryo can rupture the tube and cause severe bleeding.

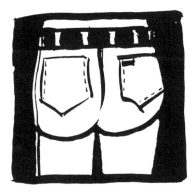

Rectum and anus

Chlamydia or gonorrhea microbes can infect the **rectum**. This can happen after anal sex with an infected partner. (Anal sex = putting the penis into a partner's rectum).

The vaginal inlet and anus are very close to each other. In women who already have Chlamydia or gonorrhea in the vaginal region, there can be direct spread of the microbes from vagina to anus.

Most people (80%) with rectal disease will have no symptoms. A few will have a rectal discharge. There may be a burning feeling around the anus.

Other symptoms

Throat

Gonorrhea microbes can infect the throat. You can get this if you perform oral sex on an infected partner.

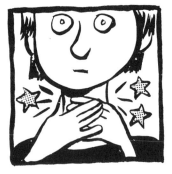

Symptoms are the same as those of any sore throat. Lab tests (see next chapter) are needed to find out if gonorrhea microbes are the cause.

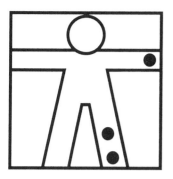

Fingers, wrist
Foot, ankle, knee

Joints
Gonorrhea microbes can spread out from the genital area by way of the blood to infect the **joints**. The joints may hurt and become swollen and tender. Often two or three joints are involved one after the other. There may be no symptoms in the genital area.

Small pustules (a pustule is a pimple that drains pus) may appear on the skin between the fingers. Pustules can also show up on the forearms or shins. The pustules are caused by gonorrhea microbes that have spread to the skin by way of the blood.

Suppose you are in a relationship that involves having sex. One day you get pain and swelling in a foot, ankle, finger, wrist, or knee joint. You didn't sprain it, and you can't explain it. What should you do? Go to a doctor or clinic and be checked for gonorrhea.

Chronic arthritis caused by Chlamydia
Chlamydia also can cause joint pain and swelling. In this case the microbes are not present in the joints. The problem is a change in the immune system caused by Chlamydia. This change causes a form of arthritis. The arthritis can last for many years. It cannot be cured with antibiotics.

SYPHILIS

One other STD caused by bacteria is syphilis. Public health workers are alarmed at the recent increase in this STD. Syphilis is hard to detect. If not treated promptly it can cause damage to major body organs. Like all STDs, syphilis is spread by intimate sexual contact. It also can spread from a pregnant woman to her fetus.

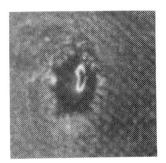

chancre

The lesion caused by syphilis microbes is called a <u>chancre</u>. A chancre is a shallow, rounded sore. Most often a chancre is not painful. It doesn't always look like a big sore. Some persons notice only a small pimple or red blotch in the area. Others don't recall any such sore.

A chancre appears about <u>four weeks</u> (10 days to 3 months) after sex with an infected person.

A chancre is **very contagious**. If you have anal sex with an infected person you can get a chancre in the buttocks area. If you perform oral sex you can get a chancre on the lips or tongue. You can even get syphilis by kissing if you kiss someone who has a chancre in the mouth area.

The chancre will always fade away after about one to five weeks. *The bad news is, that syphilis microbes remain in the body.* The person no longer feels ill. There are no signs of any disease. Even so, the person has an STD that he or she can spread to others by having sex.

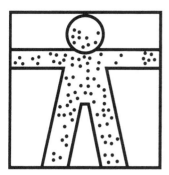
Rash due to syphilis

Rashes and patches

In most (but not all) persons, syphilis will surface again during the next 3 months. At that time a **rash** appears on the skin. The trunk, arms, and legs can all have this rash as shown. The rash may be present on the palms and soles, also. Traces of the chancre may still be present.

Inside the mouth and on the moist skin of the genitals, very contagious, **whitish patches** may appear. Small, **moist warts** can show up around the penis and vagina. The patient can feel like he or she has the flu. There is headache, fever, and swollen lymph glands. This stage of syphilis lasts for about 2-6 weeks.

Then syphilis once again appears to heal. The rashes, the patches, the warts all go away. Syphilis microbes remain in the body, where they can cause harm to vital body organs.

Late effects

Signs of the damage done may not show up until forty **years** later. There may be damage to the heart valves and to the aorta (the large blood vessel that carries blood away from the heart). There also may be damage to the nervous system and spinal cord. This can cause paralysis, trouble walking, blindness, and changes in mood or thinking ability.

HERPES-2

A common STD caused by a virus is herpes-2. At present herpes-2 is the leading cause of sores on the genitals.

Herpes-2 is cousin to a virus called herpes-1. Herpes-1 causes "cold sores" around the lips. Herpes-1 is not listed as an STD. Even so, herpes-1 can be spread during kissing or sex. Herpes-2 and herpes-1 are both **very contagious**. It is best to avoid all direct contact with any type of herpes sore.

A few days after intimate sexual contact with an infected person, that part of the skin where the herpes-2 virus entered begins to itch and redden. Soon, clusters of small blisters appear. The blisters break to form tiny sores.

Often herpes-2 sores are very painful, though they may not hurt at all. In some persons the lymph glands in the groin swell and hurt. A severe burning may be felt when passing urine. Persons with herpes-2 may get a fever and become so sick that they need to stay in bed. They may even be put in a hospital. During first-time herpes-2 infection the virus can spread to the membranes around the brain. Herpes-2 is a danger to pregnant women, because the virus can spread to the baby during birth.

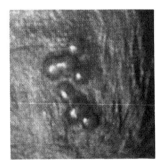

Herpes-2 blisters

How herpes-2 lesions look
The lesions caused by herpes-2 come in many shapes and sizes. How they look depends on where they are. On the skin around the genitals, herpes-2 can form tiny blisters (see left) or sores. Around the vaginal opening, herpes-2 can cause large and shallow sores. On the skin of the buttocks, legs, and thighs, herpes-2 can form large, single pimples that look a bit like acne.

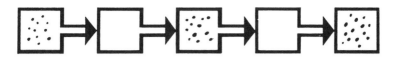

Recurrent herpes-2

After 2 to 3 weeks, herpes-2 sores go away, even when no treatment has been given. In many people, herpes-2 sores will return several weeks or months later. Often they appear in the same place where they were before. This may happen even when no further intimate sexual contact has taken place. How can this be? Even after the sores go away, herpes-2 virus stays in the body. The virus lives in nerve cells that connect to the skin. Every once in a while, the virus living in the nerve cells becomes active. It travels up a nerve fiber to the skin and causes another crop of sores.

There are no drugs that will cure herpes-2 infection. One medication will make the symptoms better (see treatment). The same drug will make the sores come back less often, and it will shorten the time that the sores stay when they do return.

Risk of cancer of the cervix
Women in whom the cervix is infected with herpes-2 virus have a problem. The risk of having cancer of the cervix later on in life is slightly increased. Such women should have a PAP test done every year to check for cancer. A PAP test is a microscope exam of scrapings taken from the cervix.

"No symptom" herpes-2
The risk of spreading herpes-2 is highest when sores are present. Even so, the sores are not always in a place where they can be seen. They may be inside the vagina or urethra. Also, persons with herpes-2 can shed the virus from their genital organs even when sores are not present. This means that a person with herpes-2 can spread the virus to others during sex even when sores are not present.

<u>Other symptoms</u>
Herpes-2 can also cause a discharge from the penis, vagina, or rectum. When the virus infects the urethra, there can be a burning feeling when passing urine. These symptoms are much like those caused by Chlamydia or gonorrhea.

Women with herpes-2 infection of the cervix can feel pain in the pelvis and in the low back area.

GENITAL WARTS (HPV)

Genital warts are caused by a virus called **Human Papilloma Virus** or **HPV** for short. "Papilloma" is a word that means "wart". HPV is a very common STD. What's worse, the rate of HPV is rising. *In many countries HPV is the most common STD!* HPV is a big problem because:

a) it is easy to spread HPV by intimate sexual contact.
b) "no symptom" HPV is common.
c) HPV can infect the cervix where it can cause a slightly increased risk of cancer.

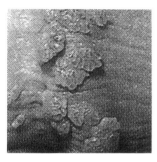

Genital Warts

How the warts look

Many patients with HPV have typical warts. The warts can be single or they can grow in clusters. They can be found on the penis, around the vagina, around the anus, or in the mouth. You can get them around the anus after anal sex with a person who has HPV. In women, anal warts also can be the result of direct spread from the vagina.

"No symptom" HPV

Many persons with HPV have warts in places where you won't see them. The warts can be inside the vagina on the cervix. In other persons with HPV there are no warts anywhere, but HPV is living in the skin. The skin where HPV is living can have a slightly strange look to it. If the suspect area is wetted with a special liquid, it will change color, marking the region affected by HPV.

Risk of cancer of the cervix and anus

Women with HPV of the cervix have an increased risk of getting cancer of the cervix later on in life. Persons with anal HPV have an increased risk of getting anal cancer.

HPV is very common. If you have HPV, this does not mean that you will get cancer of the cervix or anus. The risks are only slightly higher than normal. Women with HPV should have a PAP smear (see page 23) done every year to check for cancer of the cervix. This form of cancer is easy to treat and cure if found early.

Return of genital warts

There are a number of ways in which these warts can be removed. Treatment is discussed in a later chapter. Genital warts do come back in about 5-20% of cases. Often a return of the warts is due to a second infection from a sex partner who has HPV.

Human Immunodeficiency Virus (HIV) and AIDS

HIV is a virus that causes great damage to certain kinds of white blood cells. It infects other cells in the body, also. HIV is an STD because it is spread by intimate sexual contact. You also can get HIV by pricking yourself with a needle that has some live HIV sitting in it. This happens when the needle was used before by a person with HIV and was not sterilized afterwards.

HIV may not cause symptoms until up to **10 years (or more)** have passed. It may take that long for damage to the white blood cells to show up. White blood cells are part of the body's immune defense against infection. HIV slowly causes certain white blood cells to become weak or to die off. The body then becomes IMMUNO-DEFICIENT. It can no longer fight off infection. At this stage a person has an IMMUNODEFICIENCY SYNDROME. The syndrome is **acquired** because there was nothing wrong with the immune system to begin with. This is why the disease caused by HIV is called the :

A cquired
I mmuno-
D eficiency
S yndrome.

A person can be infected with HIV and not have AIDS. This just means that damage to the white blood cells is not yet severe. An immuno-deficient state has not yet been reached.

All persons with HIV have the virus in their blood and in their genital fluids. All can transmit the virus to others (by sex or by blood-related contact) whether or not they have AIDS!

HIV is the most feared STD because it can cause death. There is no cure for HIV or AIDS at the present time. Many persons with AIDS die because their weakened immune system fails to protect them against severe infections.

How HIV is spread

HIGH RISK
Intimate sexual contact
HIV, like any other STD, is spread by intimate sexual contact. *Semen* is fluid that a man expels from the penis during orgasm. If a man has HIV, then his semen will contain large amounts of the virus. For this reason a man with HIV is likely to infect a woman if they have unprotected **vaginal sex**. Anal sex is even more risky. **Anal sex** often causes small bruises and scrapes in the anal area. These can allow HIV to enter the body.

Spread of HIV in the other direction, from vagina to penis, or from anus to penis, is less likely, but it does happen.

The risk of spreading HIV by **oral sex** is not well known, but the risk is there. It may be harder for HIV to infect someone through the mouth than through the genitals or anus. Even so, some persons have small cuts, sores or scrapes in the mouth area. Others have damage to their gums because of gum disease. If you perform oral sex on a person with HIV, there is a chance that the virus could enter your body through such breaks in the lining of your mouth.

It is thought that the amount of HIV in normal saliva is too small to spread the infection. On the other hand, persons with gum disease or sores in the mouth can have small amounts of blood mixed with their saliva (more after brushing their teeth). If such a person with HIV performs oral sex on you, the amount of virus transferred to your genitals might be enough to infect you.

Injectable drug abuse
In persons with HIV, the virus is ALWAYS present in the blood. People who abuse injectable drugs often share needles, syringes, and the same batch of drug. If a person with HIV uses one of these, some of the live virus from his or her blood can wind up sitting in that needle, syringe or batch of drug. If you then use these things, you can inject live HIV into your body.

28

Possible methods of HIV spread due to needles, syringes, etc.
> *Self-injection with steroids (for muscle-building)*
> *Tattoos*
> *Ear piercing (or sharing pierced earrings)*
> *Friendship blood pacts*
> *Accidental needle sticks*
> *from needles thrown away in alleys or trash cans*
> *Sharing razors*

Pregnant women and breast-feeding
HIV can be spread from mother to baby while she is pregnant and when she is giving birth. HIV can be spread to the baby during breast-feeding. This is discussed in the next chapter.

LOW OR NO RISK
Getting a blood transfusion = some risk (very low)
Before 1985, HIV was sometimes spread to patients when they received blood or blood products from a donor with HIV. Enough live HIV was in the blood to transmit the disease. Today great effort is made to test blood for HIV before it is approved for use. The risk of getting HIV from a blood transfusion is now very low (but still not zero).

Giving blood or having blood drawn for tests = NO RISK
You cannot get HIV by giving blood. You cannot get HIV by having blood drawn for tests. This is because disposable needles are always used. These needles have never been used before. Young people should not fear giving blood or having blood tests for this reason.

Living with someone who has HIV = VERY LOW OR NO RISK
Although small amounts of HIV have been found in tears, feces, and saliva, HIV is not spread by casual contact. Persons living with children who have HIV are not at increased risk for getting HIV. Eating or sharing the same table or bathroom with someone who has HIV is thought to be quite safe. Doctors do advise people not to share a toothbrush or razor with a person who has HIV. During brushing, a small amount of bleeding

from the gums can occur. This can leave some HIV on the toothbrush.
Also, you should always avoid direct contact with blood that came from a
person with HIV.

Kissing

There is no evidence that HIV can be spread by kissing. As mentioned
before, there is a small amount of virus in the saliva of persons with HIV.
The amount does not appear to be large enough to infect others during
kissing.

Having said this, doctors should never say "Never!". One or both kissers
may have an open cut or sore in the mouth or on the lips. There may be
some blood in the mouth due to gum disease. In such cases, if there is
prolonged, open-mouth kissing, then one partner might transmit HIV to
the other.

SYMPTOMS

"No symptom" HIV

AIDS symptoms may not show up until months or years after the virus
first enters the body. The spread of HIV is hard to control because a
person can have HIV and not know about it for a long time. Meanwhile
he or she can be spreading HIV to others.

Symptoms of HIV

Some persons get a fever, night sweats, and swollen lymph glands
several weeks or several months after the virus first enters the body.
These symptoms last for a month or so and then go away. Many
persons never get these early symptoms.

Symptoms of AIDS
It can take months to years for the HIV virus to weaken the immune system. Only then does the person get symptoms of AIDS. These include:

> Fevers
> Weight loss (without dieting)
> Tiredness
> Diarrhea
> Swollen lymph glands
> Frequent infections

Persons with HIV that has progressed to AIDS can get pneumonia (lung infection). **PCP** or *Pneumocystis carinii* pneumonia is caused by a strange microbe that does not infect healthy persons. PCP is a leading cause of death in patients with AIDS.

HIV may damage brain cells, also. When it does the person can have trouble thinking and remembering things.

Kaposi's sarcoma
The immune system helps protect the body against certain types of cancer. When the immune system is deficient, as in AIDS, it sometimes allows cancers to take root. One cancer that AIDS patients get is called Kaposi's sarcoma. This cancer affects skin and other body organs. On the skin the tumor looks like a bruise or like a bad black and blue mark that just doesn't go away. Kaposi's sarcoma may be caused by infection by a second, as yet unknown, microbe. This cancer is one cause of death in patients with AIDS.

SYMPTOM REVIEW

Chlamydia, Gonorrhea
(burning/discharge, lower abdominal pain)

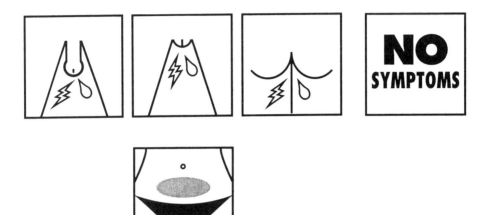

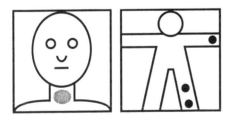

Gonorrhea when it affects organs other than the genitals: *(throat, joints)*

Syphilis
(chancre, rash)

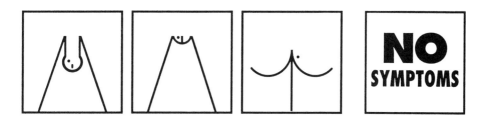

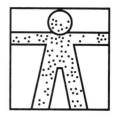

Herpes-2
(blisters/sores) These may be in places where they can't be seen, such as on the cervix. Herpes-2 also can cause discharge/burning at the penis, vagina, or rectum (not shown).

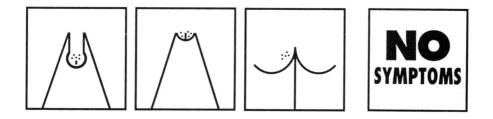

Genital warts (HPV)

(Warts) Warts may not be visible due to mild disease or because they are deep inside the vagina on the cervix.

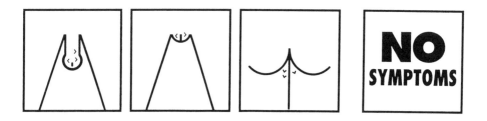

HIV infection

Most persons will have no symptoms of any kind for many months to years. For symptoms of early HIV and AIDS see pages 30-31.

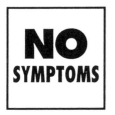

Other non-STD problems can cause symptoms similar to those shown. Refer to the pages that follow and to the Appendix section.

34

Symptoms of STDs to watch out for:

Pus-like fluid (discharge) from tip of penis, vagina, or rectum
Burning feeling when passing urine
Burning feeling or pain in the vaginal area
Need to pass urine often
Blisters, sores, or warts in the genital region
A bad smell coming from the genital region
Rash (though most rashes are NOT due to STDs!)

Review of Major Complications

Infection	Body part affected	Consequences
Chlamydia	Fallopian tubes	Blocked tubes (sterility)
Gonorrhea		Ectopic pregnancy
Syphilis	Brain	Insanity, memory/personality disorders, blindness
	Nervous system	Trouble walking, joint damage
	Heart	Damage to aorta
Herpes-2	Cervix	Slightly increased risk of cancer of the cervix
HPV (Genital warts)	Cervix, anus	Slightly increased risk of cancer of the cervix or anus
HIV	White blood cells	Immune deficiency (**AIDS**) Pneumonia (PCP) Kaposi's sarcoma DEATH
	Brain	Memory/thinking disorders

Non-STD Causes of STD Symptoms

STDs can cause:
1. Discharge or burning at the
   a. Penis
   b. Vagina
   c. Rectum
2. Pain in the lower abdomen
3. Sores/blisters/pimples/warts in the genital area

But other health problems (or non-problems) can cause these kinds of symptoms as well. Here we discuss these. The purpose is not to make you into a doctor, but to keep you from needless worry when you get a common condition that may act like an STD but is not an STD. More detail is given in the Appendix section of this book.

1a. Discharge or burning at the penis
You have a discharge coming from the tip of the penis. There is a burning feeling when passing urine. Do you have an STD? Maybe. Maybe not.

Common non-STD causes of clear or milky fluid coming from the end of the penis are:

Semen (after masturbation or after a "wet dream")
Clear fluid (after being "turned on")

Masturbation and "wet dreams"
If you masturbate to the point of orgasm, a milky fluid will be expelled from the tip of the penis. The fluid is called *semen*. Semen is a mixture of sperm and sex gland secretions. This is normal. The milky fluid is not pus. It is not due to an STD.

Sometimes a man will wake up and find milky fluid coming from the tip of the penis. This means that he dreamt of having sex. Orgasm occurred during sleep. The fluid at the tip of the penis is semen. A person may not recall such a dream. This is normal and is NOT a sign of an STD.

Clear fluid after sexual arousal
If you are "turned on" (by petting, by fondling, or by looking at sexy pictures) a small amount of clear fluid can appear at the tip of the penis. The fluid can have a slippery feel to it. The fluid is made by glands in the urethra. This is normal and is not a sign of an STD. There is no burning feeling at the tip of the penis.

Bladder or prostate infection
With this problem there may or may not be pus at the tip of the penis. You do get a burning feeling when passing urine. Also, you may feel the need to pass urine every few minutes.

The microbes that infect the bladder or prostate gland get there by coming up the urethra. Often these bacteria come from your own skin or stool. For this reason most bladder and many prostate infections are NOT due to STD microbes. These are not spread by intimate sexual contact. On the other hand, some prostate infections are due to STD microbes. All need treatment with antibiotics. Bladder infection (*cystitis*) is described more fully in Appendix 1.

STDs
With an STD, the amount of pus at the penis is greatest when you get up in the morning. As was mentioned, one of the names for Chlamydia or gonorrhea is "morning drop". Why is this so? During the day, most of the pus that forms in the urethra gets washed away when you pass urine. At night the pus keeps forming and is not washed away by urine. By the time you get up, pus has filled the urethra and shows up at the tip of the penis.

How do you know if morning fluid at the tip of the penis is due to a "wet dream" or to an STD? With an STD the fluid will show up almost every morning (and during the day). "Wet dreams" happen only once or twice a month. Also, with "wet dreams" there is no burning at the tip of the penis.

> *An STD is usually the cause if:*
>
> - BOTH burning and discharge are
>   present.
> - The discharge is worse in the
>   morning, but it is present
>   almost every morning and
>   it also shows up during the day.
> - Symptoms first appear days to
>   weeks after intimate sexual contact.

1b. Discharge or burning in the vaginal area

It is normal for there to be some amount of discharge in this area. The amount will vary during the menstrual cycle. An increase in the normal amount of discharge can be a sign of an STD. Also, burning while passing urine can be due to an STD. However, in most cases these symptoms are caused by **non-STD microbes**. You can get these other infections even if you NEVER had sex.

The most common non-STD microbes that produce discharge or burning in the vaginal area are:

Stool or skin bacteria (bladder infection)
Yeast *(Candida)*
Gardnerella

In women, the most common cause of burning while passing urine is **bladder infection** or **cystitis**. The most common cause of discharge, burning, and itching in the vaginal area is **yeast** infection (Candida).

Trichomonas is another microbe that can cause these kinds of symptoms. Trichomonas can be spread both by sex and by other means. Many doctors list this microbe as an STD.

Causes of increased discharge and burning in the vaginal region are described in Appendix 1.

Stress incontinence:
In some women a small amount of urine can be lost during coughing or giggling. The fluid is not pus and such persons do NOT have an STD.

Clear fluid after sexual arousal:
In women, also, a clear fluid can be produced by glands during sexual arousal. The fluid appears at the vaginal opening. It can have a slippery feel to it. This is normal. The fluid is not pus and is not a sign of an STD.

1c. Discharge or burning in the rectal area
These can be signs of an STD. On the other hand, fungus or yeast also can infect the anal region. When they do, they can cause a discharge or a burning feeling.

2. Pain in the lower abdomen
Microbes other than Chlamydia and gonorrhea also can infect the Fallopian tubes. Some are spread by having sex, others are not. All need treatment with antibiotics.

There are many causes of pain here besides infection of the Fallopian tubes. For example, pain in the lower abdomen can be due to one of these urgent health problems:

An inflamed appendix
A ruptured Fallopian tube
A twisted ovarian cyst

All of these problems require prompt treatment.

In most cases, though, pain in this region is due to some minor problem such as:

Constipation
Viral infection of the intestines
Ovulation (when an egg is released from the ovary)

3. Blisters, sores, pimples and warts in the genital area
Herpes-2, genital warts, and syphilis all cause this type of problem. A sore on the penis due to syphilis can look like a cut made by a zipper. You should never assume that a sore is a cut if you can't recall hurting yourself in this way.

STDs other than herpes-2 or syphilis can cause genital sores. These are described in Appendix 2.

Many causes of sores or pimples in this region are not grave. The cause may be something harmless like acne, a spider bite, heat rash, injury, or an infected pimple. These other causes are discussed in Appendix 2.

During pregnancy

Some STDs can be spread to the fetus while a woman is pregnant. Other STDs can be passed to the baby at the time of birth. For this reason, it is best to get an STD check-up as soon as you find out that you are pregnant.

First 3 months:
During this time the fetus is shielded against most STDs. We aren't sure yet about HIV. Even so, women who are pregnant and who have an STD have a higher than normal risk of miscarriage.

Mid- and late pregnancy:
After 3 months, the fetus is no longer safe from syphilis. If the mother has syphilis, then the microbes can enter the fetus by way of the blood. The baby may be born dead or have lasting damage to major body organs.

Syphilis
microbes

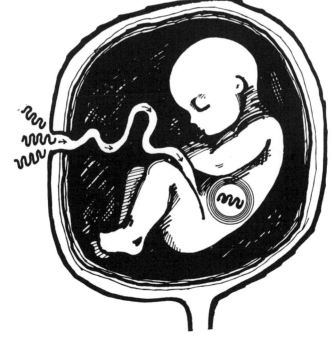

The fetus is kept shielded from STD microbes in the vagina by the *amniotic membranes*. Most people call these the "bag of waters".

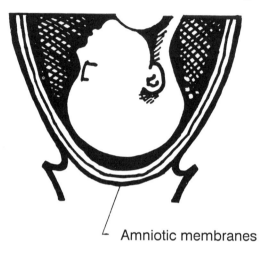

Amniotic membranes

These membranes break during labor. Now the baby is exposed. If STD microbes are present in the vagina, then the baby can get infected as it passes through the vagina during birth. The risk to the baby of getting HIV is increased at time of birth, also. Why? Often there is direct contact between the baby and the mother's blood.

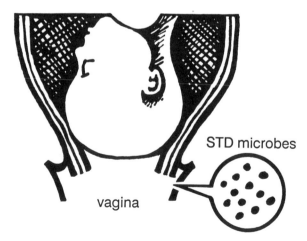

STD microbes

vagina

During and after birth

Chlamydia eye infection and pneumonia
The microbes can infect the eyes of an infant as it passes out through the vagina. If a mother has Chlamydia, then there is a 35% chance that the baby will get this eye infection. There is a 10% chance that the baby will get Chlamydia infection of the lungs.

Gonorrhea eye infection
These microbes can cause eye infection in newborn babies, also. This does not happen often, though. Why not? By law, clinics must instill antibiotic drops into the eyes of all newborns. The drops kill any gonorrhea microbes that may have gotten into the baby's eyes. Sometimes these microbes get into an infant's blood. Then they can infect and damage major body organs.

Newborn herpes
If a pregnant woman has genital herpes, there is a risk of the virus spreading to the baby during birth. In infants, herpes causes very bad disease. Many die or are left with lasting damage to the nervous system. If herpes sores are present at time of delivery, some doctors will take the baby out through the abdomen by *Caesarean section*.

Infants and children with AIDS
If a woman has HIV while pregnant, there is a 30% risk that HIV will spread to the baby before or during birth. Children with HIV often show symptoms by 2 years of age. Sometimes symptoms don't appear until 3-5 years of age. As children with HIV progress to AIDS, they can no longer fight off infections. They fail to grow. Often they die before they can become teenagers. New antiviral drugs may slow down the damage caused by HIV.

HIV and breast feeding
HIV can be spread to the infant in this manner. Mothers who know they have HIV should not breast feed their infants.

<u>Infant genital warts</u>
Infants born to mothers with HPV sometimes get warts on their sex organs or on their vocal cords. This is unusual but it may happen. It is thought that HPV spreads to the baby's genitals or mouth as the baby passes out through the vagina.

When warts form on the vocal cords, they can cause breathing problems and can be hard to get rid of.

Complications (summary)

STD complications that can affect the fetus or baby:

Chlamydia	Eye infection Pneumonia
Gonorrhea	Eye infection Damage to major body organs
Syphilis	The fetus may be born dead. Damage to many major body organs
Herpes-2	Serious nervous system infection
Genital warts *(uncommon)*	Warts on the sex organs; warts on the vocal cords (breathing problems)
HIV	AIDS in the child, which can lead to death

Lab tests

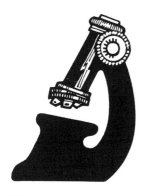

Lab tests are needed to help detect STDs. They can spot "no symptom" disease caused by Chlamydia, gonorrhea, syphilis, or HIV. When a person has symptoms, lab tests can prove that the symptoms are due to an STD and not to some other problem.

Microscope tests
Chlamydia
Gonorrhea
Herpes-2
Syphilis

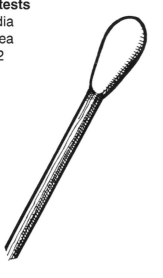

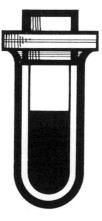

Swab tests
Chlamydia
Gonorrhea
Herpes-2

Checking the blood
Syphilis
HIV

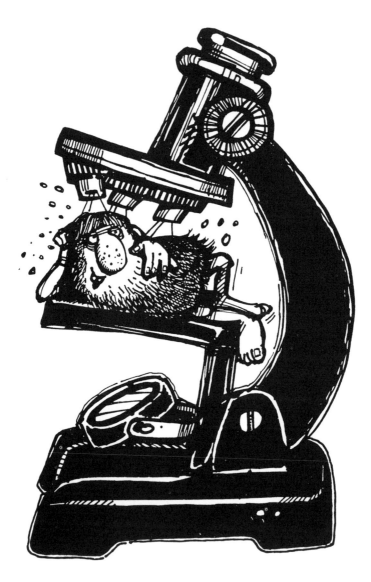

Looking under the microscope

Chlamydia:
These microbes are too small to be seen. There is a test that can be used, though. A bit of the discharge is placed in a test tube and mixed with special antibodies. These are proteins that stick only to pieces of Chlamydia and to nothing else. The antibodies are tagged with a dye that glows in the dark. They can be tagged with an enzyme, also. An enzyme is a protein that causes a chemical reaction.

The mixture of discharge + antibody + tag is then tested. If pieces of Chlamydia are present, they will be colored by the dye. This will show up under a microscope. If an enzyme tag was used, more chemicals are added to the mixture. If Chlamydia fragments were present, then the enzyme will stick to them and a chemical reaction will take place.

Gonorrhea:
A drop of the discharge is observed. Often one can see the microbes sitting inside cells.

Herpes-2:
Scrapings are taken from an opened blister or sore. The virus is too small to be seen. Herpes-2 does cause odd changes to cells. If cells in the scrapings are altered in this odd way, then herpes-2 is present.

Syphilis:
Scrapings are taken from the chancre. Syphilis microbes are hard to see but they will show up when looked at using a **"darkfield" microscope**. This uses a special light. The microbes look like tiny worms.

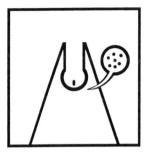

Swab tests

Most often, live Chlamydia or gonorrhea microbes will be present in the discharge. Herpes-2 virus will be living inside the blisters or sores.

Your doctor can collect some microbes by lightly rubbing a swab against the region in question.

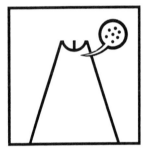

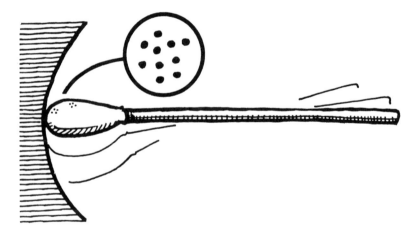

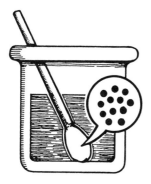

Culturing the swab

Gonorrhea:
The swab is rolled onto a jelly-like substance (agar) that contains minerals and nutrients.

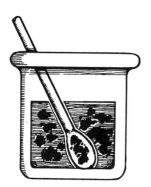

Any gonorrhea microbes present will grow and divide on the agar. Soon there will be clumps of them, enough to be seen with the naked eye.

Chlamydia or Herpes-2:
These microbes will not grow on agar, but they will infect cells. For this test, cells are kept growing in a lab dish. A bit of the discharge is placed in the dish. Any microbes present will infect the cells. One can detect their presence by staining the cells with dyes or by using other special techniques.

Checking the blood

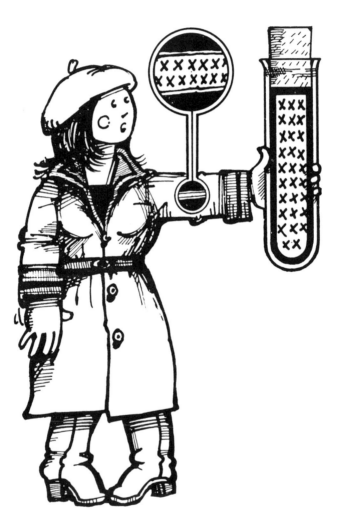

Syphilis

The body reacts to syphilis by making a special protein called *reagin*.
You can detect this protein in the blood.

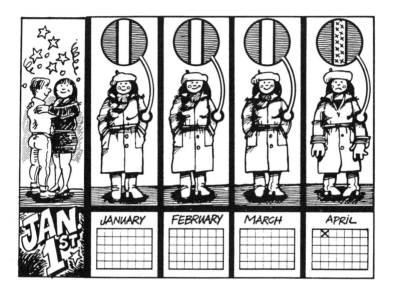

There is a 'time-lag' problem with this test. *Reagin* appears in the blood
only after a number of weeks have passed. In fact, up to three months
may go by before enough reagin is in the blood for the test to be positive.

HIV

Blood tests are used to detect HIV, also. The **ELISA** test looks for antibodies against HIV. The **Western blot** test looks for pieces of HIV in the blood.

It takes time for enough HIV antibody or HIV fragments to build up in the blood for the blood tests to turn positive. The usual time lag is 6 weeks. In some cases, 6 months (or more) may pass before the tests become positive.

Mental effects of taking an HIV blood test:

If you think you have HIV, you need to take the blood tests. Why? So you can get early treatment. This may delay or reduce the bad effects of HIV on your immune cells. Once you know you have HIV, you must avoid the risk behaviors that could spread the virus to others.

Before you go for the test you should think ahead. What if the test is positive? How will this affect you? Persons with HIV can have trouble getting health or life insurance. You may have problems getting a job (even though discrimination against persons with HIV is against the law in many regions). You might lose some of your friends. Many people are afraid of persons with HIV. They have wrong ideas about how HIV is spread.

The HIV blood test should always be done in a way that will keep the results private. You need to make sure this will be the case.

Public health clinics are very much in tune with these problems. They should counsel you BEFORE sending you for an HIV blood test. For more answers call one of the AIDS hotlines listed at the end of this book.

Blood test time lags: What they mean to you.

> If you get **syphilis**
> your blood test may not
> turn positive for up to **3 months**.
>
> If you get **HIV**,
> your blood test may not
> turn positive for up to **3-6 months (sometimes
> longer)**.

> If your partner has syphilis or HIV,
> his or her blood tests can stay normal
> for these lengths of time.

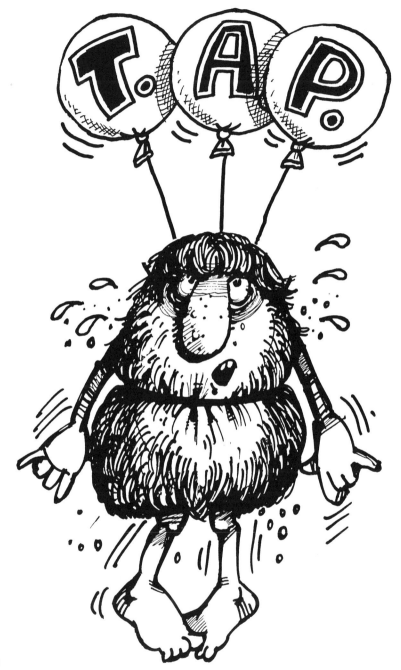

Treatment

The T.A.P. method
Your doctor or the health care team at your clinic may not talk about the "T.A.P." method. They will take three steps in treating an STD: **T**ests, **A**ntibiotics, and **P**artner notification.

TESTS

These were described in the last chapter.

ANTIBIOTICS

STDs caused by BACTERIA
Antibiotics can kill **Chlamydia**, **gonorrhea**, and **syphilis** microbes. These STDs can be fully cured if treated early. Any old antibiotic will not work. You need to be treated with the right drug and for the required length of time.

After you have been treated and cured, you do not become immune. You can get the same STD again by having sex with an infected partner.

STDs caused by VIRUSES
If you have **herpes-2**, **HPV**, or **HIV**, then you are infected with a virus. There are no drugs strong enough to kill all of the virus in your body. Viral STDs cannot be fully cured. There are drugs that can slow these microbes down and reduce the bad effects they cause.

Herpes-2 usually requires no treatment. Even so, **acyclovir** is a drug that is often quite useful. Treatment of first-time infection can make the symptoms less severe. Treatment also can make the sores return less often and for shorter time spans.

Genital warts can be treated by painting them with liquids that contain antiviral chemicals. Another method is to remove them by surgery or to destroy them by electric current or by freezing. Once you have been treated and the warts go away, HPV virus stays in the area. It is not known if such persons can still spread HPV. Most often, they probably do not.

It is not possible to cure **HIV** at present, but many promising drugs are being tested. One drug, **zidovudine (AZT)** may slow the rate of damage to the immune system.

PARTNER NOTIFICATION

As soon as you suspect that you may have an STD, stop having sex at once!

The next step is to warn your sexual partners. They need to get prompt medical help, also.

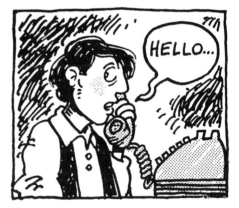

A bit of advice:
- Take your partner with you when you visit your doctor or clinic. You both can be checked and treated at the same time.
- Call your partner on the phone.

How to do it:
It may not be easy to get them to seek medical help. Your partners may try to laugh the problem off. They may ignore the dangers of having an STD. You may not know enough to give them all the facts.

One place where you can find help is your public health clinic. Here you can find trained advisers who help STD patients warn their partners. These experts do not give your name out to your partners. They do not tell them exactly when possible spread of an STD took place.

Public health clinics are too busy to give this kind of help for all STDs. When the STD is herpes-2 or genital warts, you are on your own.

In some parts of the world, there are laws about keeping results of HIV tests private. Sometimes these laws prevent public health clinics from warning partners in the case of HIV. You need to find out what the law is in your region.

Viral STDs:
For a viral STD (herpes-2, HPV, or HIV) you might think: "This can't be fully cured. Why bother warning my partners?" There are at least three reasons:

> 1) Your partners may not know that they have a viral STD. Once they know, they can take steps to stop giving it to others. Partner notification is one way to stop the spread of STDs like HIV.

> 2) In the case of HIV, there are new drugs that can slow the damage being done to the immune system. They work best if given early. To get early treatment you must know that you have the disease.

> 3) When your partner is checked out, a second, bacterial STD may be found as well. Such an STD can be treated and cured with antibiotics.

How far back to go:
This depends on the STD. The advice given below is only a rough guide. These are decisions to be made with the help of your doctor or clinic.

After you alert your PRESENT PARTNER, you should think about warning other partners from the recent past. When you get an STD, symptoms appear only after an **incubation period** has passed. You may have spread the STD to others during this incubation period.

Chlamydia, gonorrhea, herpes-2

Partners since symptoms began.
Partners from the **month** (1-4 weeks) prior to onset of symptoms.

Syphilis

Partners since symptoms began.
Partners from the **3 months** prior to a chancre
Partners from the **6 months** prior to a rash

Suppose you can't recall a chancre or rash. All you had was a positive blood test. What do you do? Take a **12-month period**, going backward from the day you were diagnosed. Warn all the partners you had during that time span.

Genital warts

Partners since symptoms began. No one knows how far to go back. There can be a 3 week to an 8 month delay from the time you get infected to the time the warts show up.

HIV

Go back to the day you think you were infected with HIV. Include all sex partners and all persons with whom you shared injectable drugs or needles from that day on. If you're not sure, go back 12 months from the day you were diagnosed. Ask your doctor for advice in this matter.

Incubation periods:
Chlamydia (burning, discharge)	*days to weeks*
Gonorrhea (burning, discharge)	*2-8 days*
Herpes-2 sores (first-time)	*2-12 days*
Syphilis chancre	*10-90 days*
Syphilis rash	*1-6 months*
Genital warts	*3 weeks to 8 months*

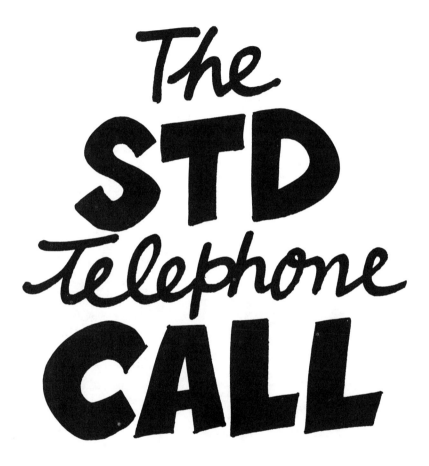

The STD Telephone CALL

63

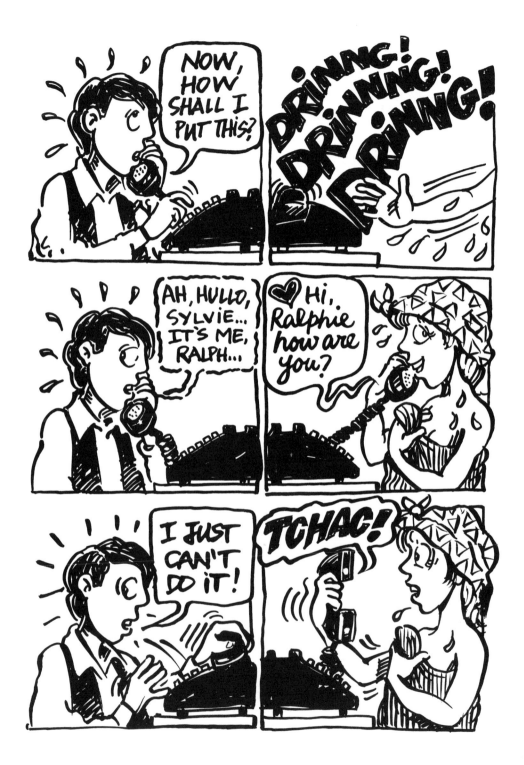

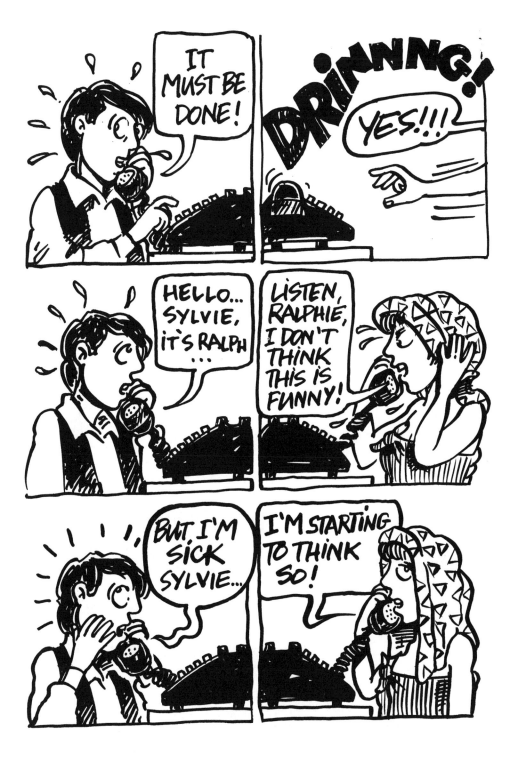

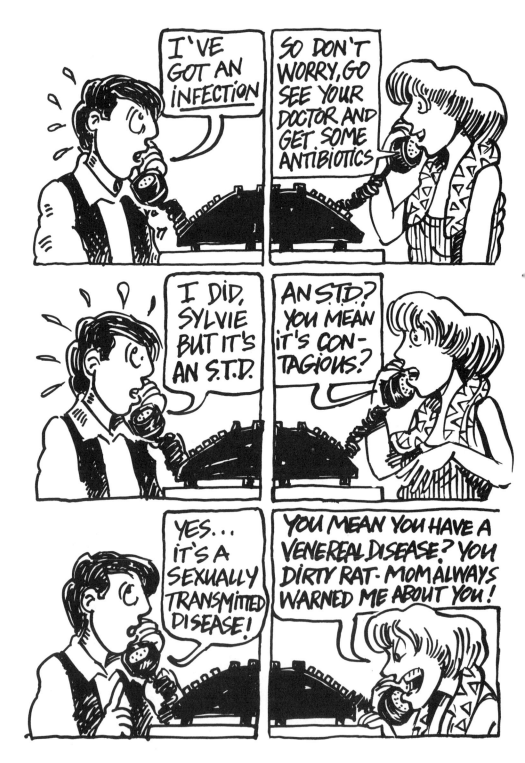

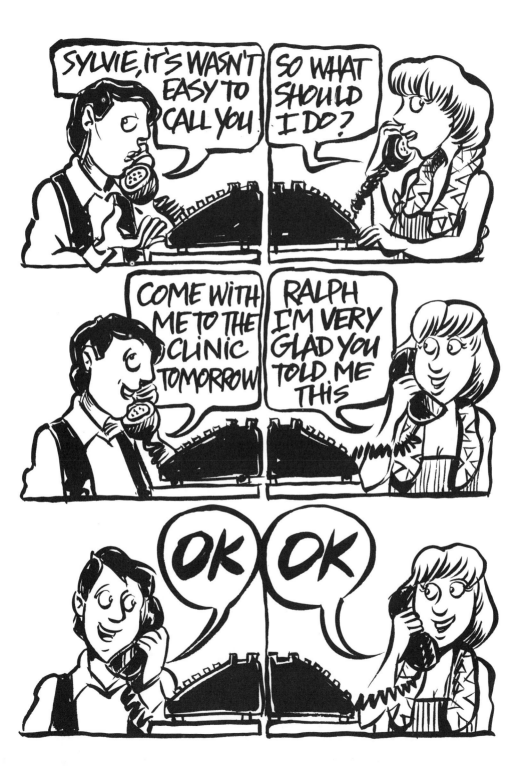

What kind of doctor to see

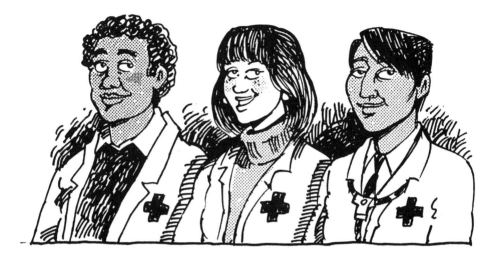

STDs can be treated by any licensed doctor. Your family doctor, your pediatrician, your internist, or your Student Health doctor can all give you the proper care.

Don't forget about your school nurse. He or she can answer your questions, check you out, and refer you for treatment if needed.

Patients sometimes go to specialists to be treated for an STD:

Gynecologist: treats problems of the female sex organs

Urologist: treats problems of the male sex organs, kidney, and bladder

Dermatologist:	treats skin problems, including all types of sores, warts, and rashes (such as those caused by herpes-2, HPV, and syphilis).
Infectious Disease Specialist:	found in clinics allied with large hospitals; often consulted to detect and treat HIV/AIDS.

Medical centers

These often schedule a weekly infectious disease clinic. Here good care for STDs can be found.

Public health clinics

Good care for STDs is offered here as well. These clinics are set up by state and local health departments. Often they hire experts in the field of STDs. Many employ persons who are trained to do partner notification. Most of the needed lab tests should be handy.

Emergency rooms:

These have their good points and their bad points. One good thing is, that you will be seen right away. This is vital. Also, for some people, an emergency room can be the only available source of health care. The bad side is, that the proper lab tests are not always close at hand. The doctor may be busy with very sick patients. There often is no follow-up care.

Time is of the essence

If you think you may have an STD, you need **prompt** medical help. Some helper in the doctor's office or clinic may try to schedule your visit three weeks (or three months) from today. Don't stand for this. Raise a fuss! If this doesn't work, look for help somewhere else.

At the doctor's office

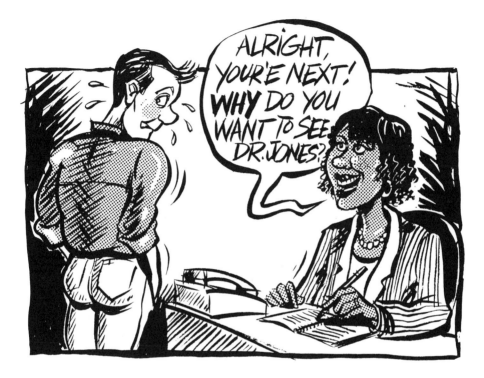

You think you may have an STD. You wind up here. What should you expect?

<u>The clerk at the counter</u>
There may be other people in the waiting room. You approach the clerk with your problem. You are embarrassed. What do you say? Consider telling the clerk that you have a burning feeling while passing urine. This is a common symptom that may or may not be caused by an STD.

With the doctor or nurse

Now you are in with the doctor or nurse. If you suspect that you may have an STD, **then say so!** Your doctor or nurse cannot always detect an STD by a simple exam. You may be questioned about your recent sexual partners. These questions are asked to learn when and how you might have become infected.

Exam for men

Your penis, scrotum, and anal area will be checked for warts and sores. Your doctor may insert a gloved finger into your rectum. This is to check your prostate gland. The prostate may be infected when there are symptoms of burning while passing urine.

After cleansing the area, a very thin swab or wire loop may be put into the opening of the urethra (this does not hurt), to sample body fluids from this region. The swab is placed into a bottle and sent to the lab for culture (see "swab test", pages 50-51).

If you have had anal sex, then say so. You may have an anal STD. Your doctor may want to obtain a swab test from there as well.

A sample of any discharge that may be present can be checked under the microscope. Your doctor will be searching for gonorrhea microbes inside cells. The discharge also can be mixed with antibodies tagged with dye or enzymes to check for Chlamydia.

Exam for women:

You will be asked to lie on a special table. This makes it easier to perform a pelvic exam. The vaginal and anal regions will be checked for warts and sores. Next, a *speculum* will be put into the vagina. This is a plastic cylinder with walls that spread apart. It allows your doctor to check the deep parts of the vagina, including the cervix. Swab tests (cultures) may then be taken:

One swab is rubbed against the inside of the cervix. A second swab is used to sample body fluids from the anal region. If there is a discharge or burning when passing urine, a third swab is used to sample the opening of the urethra.

The speculum is removed and two gloved fingers are put into the vagina. The uterus is gently rocked back and forth. This should not be painful. If it is, then the Fallopian tubes might be infected.

Both men and women
If a suspect blister or sore is present, the opened blister or sore might be scraped with a wand. The tissue obtained can be checked under a microscope for evidence of herpes-2 altered cells. The sample can be checked using a darkfield microscope to see if syphilis microbes are present.

Blood can then be drawn to test for syphilis and HIV. You should be counseled, though, before you agree to have your blood tested for HIV.

This completes the STD check-up.

Follow-up
At this point, your doctor may decide to treat you with antibiotics right away, without waiting for test results.
This happens when:

    -You have typical symptoms of Chlamydia, gonorrhea, or
        syphilis
    -Your sex partner was found to have one of these STDs

You may be treated for an STD without having the tests described. Not all labs can do these tests and they are not perfect. Sometimes STD microbes don't grow in culture, so the sample taken by the swab gives negative results. One also can miss the changes due to STDs when looking at the discharge or at scrapings from sores under a microscope.

If you had typical symptoms or if your tests are positive, you need to warn your current and recent sexual partners. Your doctor or clinic can advise you how to do this.

It's over!

Now you put on a nice smile, pass back out through the waiting room, and leave. Or is it really over? Because of time lag problems, you may need another blood test for syphilis 3 months from now. For HIV the time for a repeat test will be 6 months from now.

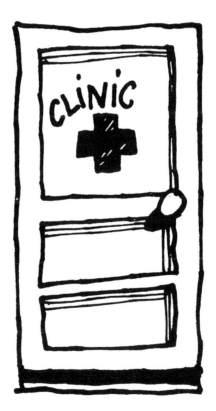

Part two

Prevention

Abstinence

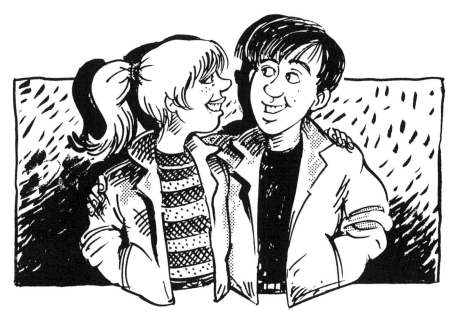

Postponing sex (abstinence)

How do you protect yourself against STDs? The most foolproof way is not to engage in sex of any kind. You and your partner abstain from sex until the time you marry. Neither you nor your partner abuse injectable drugs. Once you do marry, you stay faithful to each other. Then your risk of getting an STD will be zero or close to zero. It's that easy. Or doesn't it happen that way anymore?

Sound too tough? The game plan is to postpone sex, not to avoid sex. This strategy has a number of strong points. Having sex too soon can involve you emotionally more than you might want. These tangles and ties might wind up blocking key goals in your life such as getting a good education. Sex too soon can rob you of the chance to meet and enjoy many friends and to grow through a series of friendships. Sex too soon can distort your natural progress through your teenage years. They are a once in a lifetime experience!

If you postpone sex, you avoid the risk of someone getting pregnant when they didn't want to. It is not easy to care for a child before you yourself have had a chance to grow up.

To postpone sex does not mean to put off having boyfriends or girlfriends. There are many ways of showing your partners you like them (or love them) besides having sex. You hold hands, you caress and hug each other. You spend time together. You talk about your feelings, hopes, and dreams. This allows your relationship to develop deep roots and to mature and bloom in its own time.

Mutual monogamy (MM)
This is a less effective strategy than postponing sex. MM does have some good points, though. The game plan is this: You and your partner make a deal: You will have sex with each other, but with no one else. For MM to work, two things must be true:

1) Neither you nor your partner can have an STD at the start of your relationship.
2) Your partner must be trustworthy. Otherwise, he or she can get an STD from someone else while your relationship is still going on.

Are you sure that your partner doesn't have an STD right now? Maybe he or she has an STD but doesn't know it. Remember that "no symptom" STDs are common. Remember that there is a time lag before a blood test for syphilis or HIV turns positive.

Know your partner well before you decide to have sex
Suppose your partner
  -had sex with many persons in the past.
  -is having sex with many persons now.
  -abused injectable drugs in the past.
  -is abusing injectable drugs now.

This person is at high risk for having an STD right now. This person is at high risk for getting an STD in the near future.

People have secrets. People are not always what they seem to be. Welcome to the real world! How can you find out these sorts of things about your partner? You don't need to hire a detective or to check police records. The best strategy is to TAKE YOUR TIME. Get to know your partner's friends and relatives. Talk to people. Find out who your partner is before you commit yourself to having sex. Don't have sex with people you "fall in love with" on trips or vacations. Don't have sex with strangers!

Meanwhile, talk, talk, talk to your partner! Don't be afraid to discuss health and other things that mean a lot to you, such as your hopes and dreams for the future.

Danger of using drugs
Using drugs is risky for many reasons. Here we list only those dangers that pertain to STDs.

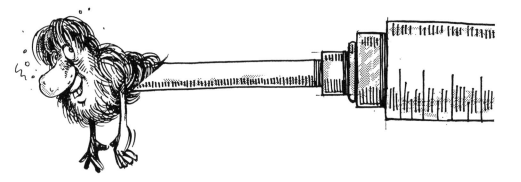

Danger ONE: Contaminated drug equipment:
Suppose you inject yourself with drugs. You happen to use a needle, syringe, or drug liquid that was used beforehand by someone with HIV or hepatitis (see Appendix 5). Virus from that person's blood might be in the drug equipment that you just used. You may have just shot HIV or hepatitis virus into your body!

Danger TWO: Impaired judgement
Drugs, most often alcohol, sometimes are used by a person to help seduce a partner. Drugs such as alcohol, marijuana, LSD, "ecstasy", cocaine, or heroin, can cloud your thinking. They can impair your ability to make good decisions. You will then be making a decision (to have sex, for instance) when you can't think clearly about the possible consequences.

Danger THREE: Social circle

Persons who abused injectable drugs in the past or who are abusing drugs now are at high risk for having an STD by way of contaminated drug equipment or by way of having sex with many partners. Some have many, many sex partners because they trade sex for money in order to buy drugs.

If you start to abuse injectable drugs, then these are the kinds of people who will wind up being your "friends". One day you may have intimate sexual contact with them. One day you might share a needle, syringe, or batch of drug with them.

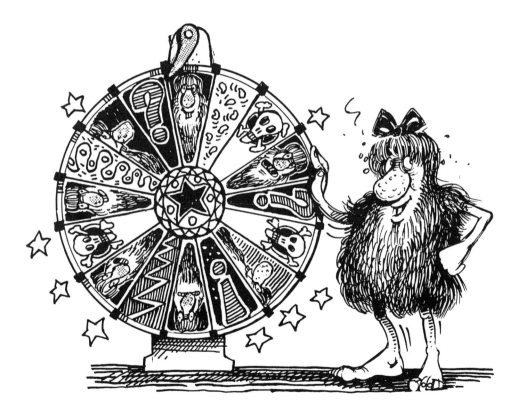

Latex Condoms

Latex condoms
If you decide to have sex with your partner, make sure you ALWAYS use a latex condom. A latex condom gives you good (but not perfect) protection against getting **gonorrhea, Chlamydia,** or **HIV**. A latex condom will only protect you some of the time against **herpes-2, syphilis, or genital warts.** Why? The sores or warts that these microbes cause can be outside of the area covered by a condom.

If you suspect or know your partner has HIV, you should never have sex with that person, even if you are protected by a condom. The risk of getting HIV may be reduced, but it is still there, and you are risking your life.

The big problem with latex condoms
People don't use them EVERY time. Why not?

You're afraid to go out and buy one at the drug store or super market.
> Don't be scared of buying a latex condom. Be more afraid of what might happen if you don't use one!

You want to use a condom, but you don't have one handy.
> You cannot always foresee when you will decide to have sex. If there is any chance for this, then you should keep a latex condom with you on that day. A woman should not assume that her partner will have a latex condom with him. On that day, she should keep one in her purse.

You want to use a condom, but don't know how.

Many classes on sex education teach students the right way to use latex condoms. Some tips are:

-Never use an oil-based lubricant such as baby oil or Vaseline. These can weaken latex condoms and cause them to break. Use a water-based lubricant instead.

-Before you roll the condom on, pinch the end so as to leave a little pouch at the tip. Keep the pouch pinched while you roll the condom on. The pouch will help keep the condom from breaking during use. Also, the pouch will collect any semen that is expelled.

-When you are ready to pull out of the vagina, put your fingers around the free end of the condom at the root of the penis. Pull the condom out with the penis so that it doesn't get left behind.

-If you want to have sex a second time, don't try to use the same condom again! Go to the bathroom. Take the condom off. Wash your genitals with soapy water. Dry them. Put on a new condom when you are ready to go again.

You want to use a condom, but your partner thinks it's "not romantic"

Romance is a state of mind and of the imagination. If your partner really cares about you, your health, and your safety, then he or she will not object if you use a condom. In fact, your partner should insist that you use one.

Other words for condom: 　　　　*Safe* 　　　　*Rubber* 　　　　*Prophylactic*

<u>Latex vs. animal skin</u>
Most condoms sold today are made of latex plastic. Latex condoms are quite good at stopping passage of STD microbes, even those that are viruses.

Condoms made of animal "skin" (sheep gut) also are sold. Animal skin condoms are not as good as latex condoms, because often they have tiny holes in them. These can allow small STD microbes (like HIV) to slip by.

Latex condoms are not perfect, either. Sometimes there are small holes in them because of problems in the way they are made.

<u>Nonoxynol-9:</u>
This is a chemical that kills sperm. It comes as a foam that is put into the vagina using a small plunger, or it can be in a vaginal tablet or sponge. Some condoms come packaged in a lubricant that contains nonoxynol-9.

Nonoxynol-9 can kill several kinds of STD microbes. Even so, it will not keep you from getting an STD if used alone. It may stop you from getting an STD if you also are using a latex condom. If you have used lots of nonoxynol-9, it might kill any STD microbes that managed to get through or around the condom. The small amount of nonoxynol-9 that is present in condom lubricants may not do much good.

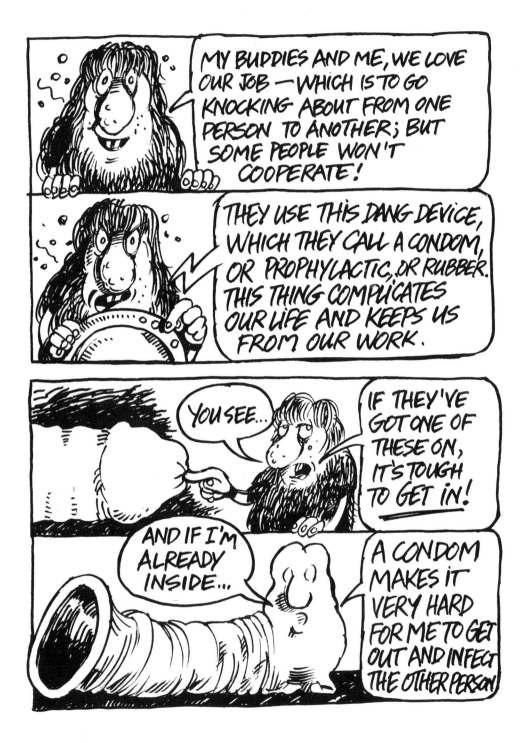

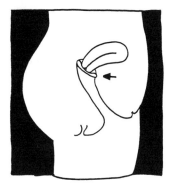

Diaphragm

A diaphragm (arrow) covers the cervix deep inside the vagina. It does not cover the rest of the vaginal lining. Using a diaphragm is NOT a good way to protect yourself against STDs.

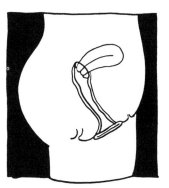

Female Condom

This is new. It is a sheath that the woman inserts into the vagina before having sex. There is an inside ring that expands around the cervix, and an outside ring that covers the vaginal inlet. The sheath does protect the entire vaginal lining as well as the cervix. Use of the female condom may turn out to be a fairly good way to protect yourself against many STDs. This is still being studied. The female condom allows a woman to take the matter of STD protection into her own hands.

Popular methods of STD prevention that don't work:

-Passing urine or washing the penis after sex

-Douching after sex

-Using antibiotic creams or ointments

Will taking an antibiotic right before or after sex prevent you from getting gonorrhea, Chlamydia, or syphilis?

People who trade sex for money tried this method years ago. They thought that if they took a pill of penicillin every day, then they would be safe from getting gonorrhea. They were wrong! They still got gonorrhea because there was not enough antibiotic in their bodies to kill the microbes. What's worse, the microbes became immune to penicillin. Now gonorrhea is much harder to cure than it was 20 years ago.

There are problems with this "preventive" approach. You may take the wrong antibiotic. You may take too small an amount of the right antibiotic. You may take the right amount of the right antibiotic, but not for a long enough period. In all of these cases, you may kill most of the STD microbes, but not all of them. Symptoms may never appear, but a "no symptom" STD will remain in your body.

Antibiotics don't work at all against the viral STDs. You can take huge amounts before having sex. If your partner has herpes-2, genital warts, or HIV, antibiotics will not keep you from getting these STDs.

Prevention of HIV after possible exposure

By accident, health care workers sometimes do stick themselves with a needle that was used on a patient with HIV. In such cases, an experimental treatment is to take an antiviral drug for some time afterwards. The hope is, that you might prevent any HIV that entered the body from surviving. We don't know yet if this works. Meanwhile, better methods of disposing of used needles are being designed.

Immunity and vaccines

There is no such thing as "immunity" to an STD. If you get a bacterial STD and are cured by antibiotics, you can catch the same STD again if you have sex with another infected partner.

At this time, there is no effective vaccine against any of the STDs. Some vaccines against HIV are being tested, but none are yet ready for regular use in humans.

There is a vaccine against one type of hepatitis (type B). If you are at high risk for getting an STD, then you, also, are at high risk for getting hepatitis (see Appendix 5). In such cases, you should get this vaccine.

Decision making

Many persons have sex or take drugs even though they never decided ahead of time that they wanted to. Why? Peer pressure, mostly. You slide into a situation which leads you to having sex or taking drugs. Sometimes it isn't a question of sliding but of being pushed. You simply let someone else's will take you over. You let yourself get "talked into" it.

You can read this book. You can listen to the advice of your parents, teachers, counselors, and friends. The decision to have sex now or to postpone sex is up to you. If you already are having sex now, then you have other decisions to make. Who will you have sex with? Will you insist that you and your partner practice mutual monogamy? Will you protect yourself always by insisting that a latex condom be used? Will you stop having sex now and postpone sex once again?

Consequences
Are you a good decision maker? To be a good at this, you need to look at the consequences of your decisions. These can be good or bad. Let's take a few decisions:

POSTPONE SEX OR HAVE IT NOW?

You are thinking of having sex with your partner. You have not been sexually active. You think ahead of the consequences, both good and bad. Imagine that you did have sex. What would the consequences be?

Good
a) Curiosity, independence, self-awareness
> You wanted to find out what sex is like, and now you know. You wanted to feel more independent and grown up, and now you do. You weren't sure you could go through with having sex. Now you know.

b) Getting closer to your partner

You wanted to feel closer to your partner. You wanted your partner to feel closer to you. Now that you have had sex, you feel closer, and you hope that he (she) does, also.

c) Popularity

All your friends seemed to be having sex and talking about it. You always used to feel left out. Now maybe you'll be one of the crowd (or will you?).

d) Earning money

You used sex to earn money. You needed money and wanted to buy certain things very badly. Now you have the money and can buy them.

Bad

a) Being vulnerable

You may become more emotionally involved with your partner than before. This will make you more vulnerable to his (her) actions and desires. You may be hurt deeply if that person decides to leave you, or if you find out that he (she) has other emotional ties. Sometimes, after two people have sex, one of them becomes afraid of the emotional ties that start to form and breaks off the relationship.

b) Playing games

Having sex might have been only a game for your partner. Now that he (she) has "seduced" you, your partner may no longer be interested in you.

c) Unwanted pregnancy

There is a risk of pregnancy and the problem of caring for an unwanted child. For either a woman or a man, a pregnancy at the wrong time can have a very bad effect on career and educational plans. You will be responsible for, and attached to, a child you did not want. You may have to pay child support. You say that you don't have to worry about this because you used an effective means of birth control? Maybe. But as a good decision maker, you should think ahead: "But what if a child were to result?" What would I do then? What would my partner do? How would this affect me?

d) STDs

If you have studied this book, then you should now know much about STDs and the consequences that can result.

Alternatives

A smart decision maker will always fully evaluate the consequences of the alternative choices before making a decision: For example, you might want to have sex primarily because you want to find out what sex is like. The alternative, not having sex now, would mean postponing this knowledge. However, having sex with each person is different. And if you have sex now, when you are not ready and with a person who really doesn't mean much to you, your first encounter with sex might not really give you much useful information about the possibilities of sex combined with real love.

You might want to have sex because all of your friends are pushing you into it, telling you that you need to have sex before you can become a "real man" or a "real woman". The alternative is not to have sex now because you are not ready, and because the right person for you isn't there.

Maybe you want your partner to feel closer to you. As noted above, having sex too soon can sometimes make an open relationship more confining and can scare people into breaking it off. The alternative strategy, to postpone sex, can allow your relationship to grow without the pressure of having sex.

You might want to have sex because you need money. The alternatives are to get the help you need from social agencies in your area (or to get a job).

DECISIONS FOR THOSE WHO ARE ALREADY HAVING SEX

MUTUAL MONOGAMY, YES OR NO?

You and your partner made the decision to have sex. Now you must decide whether you will make a deal to engage in mutual monogamy. What would be the good and the bad consequences?

Good

a) Low risk of STDs

Your risk of getting an STD would be lower.

b) You are making a commitment to each other

You are saying that your relationship is very important to both of you. It is so important, that you are willing to give up some freedom for it.

c) Protecting your relationship

Having sex with others might risk tearing your relationship apart because of jealousy.

Bad

a) Limiting your opportunities

Once you have entered into a mutual monogamy deal, you do give up some freedoms. You can still see and enjoy other persons, but not to the point of having sex with them.

Alternatives

The alternative decision is NOT to choose mutual monogamy. This means that you make no commitment to each other. Both of you can have sex with others during your relationship. You will not be kept back from fully exploring the possibilities of sex with other persons.

You need to ask, "What is the benefit of being able to have sex with others?". Having sex with others may have a bad effect on your main relationship, because neither of you will be making an effort or giving anything up. Your risk of getting an STD will be higher.

HAVING SEX WITH A STRANGER, YES OR NO?

You meet him or her at a party or on vacation. You dance the night away. You like the way s(he) moves. It seems you can talk to each other for hours without getting bored. You really don't know anything about him (her), but you know you are "in love".

Good
a) Having sex will allow you to fulfill your romantic fantasy of the moment.

b) Having sex may help you keep this wonderful new partner and make him (her) more interested in you (or will it?).

c) Maybe you'll never see him (her) again. This is your one chance to know what true love is really like.

d) You'll probably never see him (her) again. There will be no strings attached to your relationship.

e) Since you and your stranger don't have the same friends, your friends won't know that you had sex together.

Bad
a) You don't know this person at all. He (she) may be a phony, a drug addict, a liar, or a criminal. He (she) may not be any of these, but, after getting to know him (her) for even a week or two, you might find out that he (she) is really a selfish, unfeeling, clod. This wouldn't be bad, except now you've had sex with this person!

b) This charming partner may be one who abuses injectable drugs or who has many sex partners. His (her) risk of having an STD might be high. He (she) might have an STD right now and not know it.

c) If your stranger finds out that he (she) has an STD, he (she) may not inform you, either because he (she) doesn't care, or because he (she) won't be able to get in touch with you.

Alternatives
The alternative is to enjoy that wonderful evening or vacation with the romantic stranger, but not to have sex. Go everywhere with him (her). But don't have sex. Call them the next day. (You might be surprised by who answers the phone). See him (her) again, and again. If you're on vacation and have to go your own ways, write. Find out about his (her) parents and friends. Talk to them about your wonderful stranger, who will then no longer be a stranger. Let your relationship grow. Some of the nicest friendships that turned into romances started out among pen pals. Postpone sex.

TO USE A LATEX CONDOM EVERY TIME, YES OR NO?

You and your partner have made the decision to have sex. One of you is already using some form of birth control, so you are not very worried about pregnancy. You are considering using a condom anyway because you're afraid of getting an STD.

Good
You will protect yourself against getting an STD, at least partially, by using a latex condom.

Bad
Your partner may think you're too picky or a worry wart. You may not have a condom handy and you really don't want to miss out on having sex. You know that a condom does not offer perfect protection against STDs. You only live once, so, what the heck.

Alternatives
The alternatives are not to use a latex condom, and to run an increased risk of getting an STD. You may decide to use a condom only when you have sex with a stranger or other "high risk" person. On the other hand, you can't be sure that your present partner doesn't have (or won't get) an STD. Some of the nicest people have STDs, including HIV.

By the way, if you know or suspect that a person has HIV, you should never have sex with them, even if you are protected by a condom. The risk of getting HIV may be fairly low, but you are risking your life.

RETURNING TO ABSTINENCE, YES OR NO?

You wanted to see what sex was like. Now you know. You've had several relationships, and none of them really worked out very well. You're worried that you may not be on the right track in life. You are considering going back to the way you once were. You want to postpone sex once more. Can you ever go back?

Good

Of course you can! And postponing sex once more does not mean that you have to give up having relationships. You may find that you enjoy your boyfriends or girlfriends now more than before. Now that you have stopped having sex, you are talking more and sharing more feelings. Your risk of getting an STD will again be very low, if not zero.

Bad

You may feel that you can't get close to your partners unless they have sex. You may be afraid that you might lose a partner or be unpopular unless you have sex. Your new partners may know you had sex before with others, and resent it that now you won't have sex with them.

Alternatives

The alternative is to keep on having sex, with good and bad consequences as was already described.

How to say "NO!" when you don't want to

One very bad situation is when you don't really want to have sex, but you let yourself be talked into it.

Are you afraid that, if you say "NO",

then your partner will no longer like you?
then your partner will leave you?
then you won't be popular?
then you'll be considered square?
then you'll be giving in to your parents and their
point of view?

Some people just don't know how to say "NO". A famous psychologist, Dr. Irene Kassorla, in her book, <u>GO FOR IT</u> describes six steps that you can use to deliver a warm but firm "NO". The following is adapted from Dr. Kassorla's book:

Step 1: Stop being a child
You are almost an adult now. You don't need approval from everybody. You can say no and you won't be spanked... You won't lose approval.

Step 2: Rule out negotiations
By stating your "NO" in a brief and firm way, you will silently communicate, "I have spoken. This is not open to negotiation". Your friendliness shows that you are completely self assured, and your firmness and being brief about it signals that the issue is closed.

Step 3: Face the other person directly
When you are saying "NO" watch your body language. Look the other person straight in the eye as you talk. If your subtle gestures suggest that you feel awkward or lack confidence, then the other person will pick up this clue and not believe you.

Step 4: Don't give explanations

When you give reasons for your decision, you are implying that your decision needs justification. A long explanation raises false hopes and suggests that you may be feeling guilty and could be persuaded to reverse your decision. You are a responsible person and you don't have to defend nor prove your reasons.

Step 5: Allow yourself a time-out period to think it over

Even if you are a terrific decision maker, there will be times when you are unsure about your response and will need a few days to decide. Act confident when you tell your partner that "I want to think this over. I'll get back to you soon".

Don't be pressured into an immediate "YES" or "NO" before you are ready. Take as much time as you need to arrive at a decision that you can live with.

Step 6: Surround your "NO" with positives

First, state your honest positives to your partner. Then sandwich in a short "NO", and then close with one more honest positive. An example of this might be as follows:

Positive #1:	I'm so pleased that you want to share something so meaningful and personal with me.
Positive #2:	Our relationship is really important to me.
Positive #3.	My good feelings for you will go on forever.
Your "NO" Message:	**I just am not ready to have sex at this time.**
Positive #4.	I value you so much, I don't want anything to interfere with our loving feelings.

Then add yet another positive by putting your arm around your friend, offering some alternative suggestions, if you can. Then move on to a conversation about something else.

(Adapted with permission from GO FOR IT, by Irene Kassorla, Delacorte Press, New York, 1984).

Part three

Case Reports

Spring Break

Ralph had just come back from spring break. He had traveled WEST to think, to paint, to live it up, and just "fool around". Yesterday he had come back home. Last night, all of his friends, and Sylvie, his "steady" girlfriend, had thrown him a big "Welcome home!" party.

In the morning when Ralph woke up he felt something funny. He looked down and noticed that he had signs of Chlamydia or gonorrhea (and leaked and burned it did!). What should he do? Ralph found the phone number of a urologist and called to set up a visit. The clerk at the office told Ralph that doctor could see him, but only 3 weeks from now!

After several minutes of searching (through the telephone book), Ralph came upon a listing that read "PUBLIC HEALTH CLINIC". Yes, it was open. Yes, they could see him right away.

The clinic was in a modern office building. The staff were all pleasant and relaxed. The other patients in the waiting room appeared to be very normal. No one looked nervous or shy.

Ralph was taken to see the doctor. Ralph told her the whole story. The only person he had sex with in the recent past was a girl named Linda. Five days earlier, while still far from home, Ralph had met Linda in a city library. It was love at first sight, so he and Linda made a night of it. Since he got back, on the night of his "Welcome Home!" party, Ralph had sex with his steady girlfriend, Sylvie, also.

The doctor examined Ralph. Using a swab, she took a sample of his discharge and sent if off to the lab. The lab people looked at the discharge under a microscope for gonorrhea microbes. They mixed a sample with antibodies against Chlamydia, also. Both of these tests were negative. The swab was placed in a bottle filled with agar and sent off for culture. Some blood was drawn to check for syphilis.

Because Ralph had typical STD symptoms and recent sexual contact, the doctor decided to treat him even though his first lab tests were negative. The doctor prescribed two antibiotics; one to treat gonorrhea and one to treat Chlamydia. The doctor advised Ralph to call Linda and tell her that she probably had an STD. Also, the doctor advised him to call Sylvie. Ralph may have spread his STD to Sylvie when they had sex after he returned from his trip.

Ralph didn't know Linda very well, but he had her phone number and address. He asked the public health clinic staff to contact her. Ralph didn't blame Linda. He figured Linda didn't know that she had an STD. Ralph knew that "no symptom" Chlamydia or gonorrhea can occur often. Ralph called Sylvie himself and explained the problem. The next morning they both came to the public health clinic. Sylvie had no symptoms. Her swab culture tests for gonorrhea would turn out to be negative. Even so, the doctors decided to treat her with antibiotics.

The day after Ralph was treated, his burning and discharge went away. Ralph phoned the clinic for follow up. Yes, it was an STD. In the sample of discharge that had been sent for culture, gonorrhea microbes were now growing! Ralph and Sylvie both returned to the clinic a few more times. One week later they came for a follow-up visit. Three months later they had repeat blood tests for syphilis (because of the time lag effect).

Both Ralph and Sylvie were counseled about what they might expect from taking an HIV blood test. They decided to have the test. Because of the time-lag problem they had one test now and a repeat test six months later. Both turned out to be negative.

Sylvie didn't like the fact that Ralph had sex with another woman. Even so, Ralph did have the courage to tell Sylvie that she was at risk for an STD. Ralph and Sylvie talked, and she forgave him. They stayed together. Ralph and Sylvie made a deal. They would have sex only with each other until they were married or until they decided to split apart. They lived happily forever after (or at least for a while).

Party

Jinotta was in a good mood. In June she would finish high school. Jinotta was working part time at a large food store. After graduation, the boss promised Jinotta that she would be assistant manager.

Now it was still March. Carmen, Jinotta's best friend, made plans to celebrate their last year of high school. "Let's get together with all of our friends and have a party!" It would be a chance to listen to records, watch horror movies on the video, fill up on junk food, and talk.

The morning of the party, Jinotta went to the store to buy supplies. She was famous for her party dip: canned salmon, cream cheese, mayo, chives, and smoke flavoring. That evening, Jinotta was walking up to the door of Carmen's house. What she saw surprised her. Usually Carmen's parents were very strict. They never allowed Carmen to stay out late. They kept a very close eye on Carmen's friends. Tonight all the windows were open. Carmen's house was full of rowdy people whom Jinotta hardly knew. "Hey, welcome", Carmen greeted her from an upstairs window. "Guess what? My parents went to visit my cousins for a few days. We've got the whole place to ourselves!".

At first Jinotta had a great time. She got to talk to a lot of her old friends. She met some neat new people. For instance, there was Jerome, a friend of Carmen's brother. Jerome looked and talked like he came from some other place. He had great plans. He knew what he wanted out of life. Jerome dressed well. He had smooth lines. Jerome told Jinotta that she was like no other girl he ever knew. Jinotta got mad when she saw Denise hanging around Jerome like a jealous hen, always brushing up against him. People were dancing, talking, drinking beer, and smoking joints.

Jinotta remembered talking to Jerome, and then four people going upstairs to one of the bedrooms to "listen to some music". She remembered having sex, and not knowing when it was over.

The next morning, Jinotta felt a bit empty. She had not been in control last night. How stupid of her! Carmen was happy, though. What a great party! Everybody at school was talking about it. Well, "Chalk it up to experience!", Jinotta thought.

Six weeks later, Jinotta began throwing up in the morning. She started to feel dizzy and tired. Jinotta wasn't surprised when the pregnancy test came back positive. After talking with her counselor, Jinotta decided that she would put the baby up for adoption. Jinotta felt somewhat relieved at this point. Yes, her life was changed, but it would all get back on track again next year. She could go back and finish school, and then go on to her new job and career.

Then Jinotta's doctor called to tell her that a routine prenatal blood test for syphilis had turned up positive. "We can treat and cure you for sure," the doctor told Jinotta, "Your fetus should be cured, also. It's a good thing we caught this right away."

Jinotta was a fighter. She took comfort in the fact that her syphilis had been found and treated early. Jinotta thought that her baby would be O.K. After several weeks her normal good spirits returned.

A few months later, Jinotta's repeat blood test for syphilis showed very low levels of reagin. This was good news. It meant that her syphilis had been cured.

Jinotta was relieved. She would go on, but things would be different. Her life had been changed during one evening in March by actions she had never planned or thought about in advance.

Macho Man

Henry was a macho man. Having sex with each new woman was a challenge. It made him feel strong and gave him a sense of self worth. Henry knew about STDs and he knew about the risk of getting someone pregnant. Henry had tried using a latex condom once or twice, but he never had learned how to use it right. He had fumbled with it in the dark and hadn't known which way to put it on. Never again! No more condoms for this macho man! Since that time, Henry never carried latex condoms with him. If someone brought up the subject he would say, "No way! That would be like taking a shower with a raincoat on!".

Henry went through a lot of girlfriends. This was because he really didn't have much to say to a woman after he had gotten her into bed. Henry didn't much like talking to women anyway.

Henry had contracted an STD more than once. "It goes with the life style", he thought. Once he developed little warts on his genitals. His physician told him he had genital warts, or HPV. Henry got treated but never bothered to inform his sexual partners. That would be too "strange". Another time, Henry got herpes. Since then, a few times a year, he would notice painful blisters in his genital area. They would go away on their own after several weeks.

Then Henry met Sarah. Sarah was different. Sarah knew how to make her own clothes. She knew how to fix cars. She was good in math and was applying for a good job in a bank. Henry fell in love with Sarah. They were engaged to be married.

At first Sarah didn't want to have sex before marriage, but then changed her mind. When the subject of using a condom came up, Henry kept making excuses. He told Sarah that there was no reason to need one. There was no way he could have an STD.

Two weeks after Sarah and Henry did have sex, Sarah got a bad case of herpes. Painful blisters appeared in her genital area. She got a fever and swollen lymph glands. It was painful for Sarah to urinate. She developed bad headaches which her doctor told her might be an early sign of herpes meningitis. Her doctor treated her with acyclovir. A month later the sores came back in the same place. Sarah also got genital warts. These she had to get removed by surgery.

Sarah called off her marriage to Henry, the Macho Man. Why? Was it because she got two STDs from him?. Or because Henry had not been honest with her? Because Henry didn't care enough to warn her about his STDs and take measures to protect her?

Time bomb

Keisha and Jarmaine had known each other since first grade. They were the best of friends. Somehow they always knew that they would eventually get married. In high school Keisha and Jarmaine began going with each other. After 3 years they decided that they would have sex. They learned about STDs in school. Because they were careful people who made plans in advance, they decided that they would always use a condom whenever they had sex. During senior year in high school, Jarmaine asked Keisha to marry him. Keisha didn't wait for a second before she said yes.

Everything was coming together for Jarmaine. His grades were the best, and his basketball team was in the state finals. Jarmaine was applying to join the Navy. He wanted to get more training in electronics and computers. One day he hoped to be a computer systems analyst or start his own software company.

Jarmaine received a call from the Navy. He was to report to base to the health officer. The news from the doctor was shocking. His routine blood test for HIV turned out to be positive! The Navy was turning him down for health reasons!

How could this be? Jarmaine hadn't had sex with anyone except Keisha. He was sure that Keisha hadn't had sex with anyone else, either. Besides, he always had used a condom when having sex with her. Then he remembered his freshman year in high school. He had tried drugs. He remembered injecting heroin into his veins with a group of friends at an abandoned house. Jarmaine hadn't liked it. He had decided quickly that drugs just weren't for him. That must have been it! It was the only way he could have gotten HIV.

Keisha was tested the next week. Her HIV test was negative.

How did this all end?

a) Keisha was horrified at the risk of getting AIDS. She told Jarmaine to take a hike. Jarmaine began to get symptoms of AIDS. Despite the best medical care, he developed pneumonia, weight loss, and diarrhea. He died two years later.

b) Keisha was horrified at the risk of getting AIDS. She told Jarmaine to take a hike. Jarmaine became a spokesman for various AIDS groups around the city to tell young persons about the dangers of drugs. He still has no symptoms.

c) Keisha decided to stay by her man. They got married anyway. They decided that they would have no sex for the time being. They adopted two beautiful children. In the year 2000, a cure for HIV was finally discovered. Jarmaine took the cure and it was successful. They had three more children of their own and lived to a ripe old age.

Part four

Appendices

APPENDIX 1

Other causes of burning and increased discharge
in the vaginal area

Microbes other than Chlamydia, gonorrhea or herpes-2 often cause these symptoms. The most common are:

1. **Stool or skin bacteria** (causing **cystitis**)
2. **Candida** (a yeast)
3. **Trichomonas** (a protozoan)
4. **Gardnerella** (a bacterium)

CYSTITIS

Bacteria from the stool or skin can be spread (by wiping) from the anus to the opening of the urethra (the tube that takes urine from the bladder to the outside). The microbes can then move up the urethra into the bladder to cause infection there. This is called **cystitis**. This happens more often in women than in men. Why? In women the urethra is short. Wiping from back to front after passing stool may increase the risk of getting cystitis.

Symptoms are like those seen with Chlamydia or gonorrhea. The microbes in the urine inflame the urethra. As a result there is a burning feeling when passing urine. It is common to feel the need to pass urine often (for instance, every 15 minutes). It may be hard to hold the urine back. The microbes in the bladder can spread to the kidneys. Then patients can feel pain in the back. There can be fever and chills.

T.A.P. for CYSTITIS

<u>Tests</u>:
Under the microscope you can often see white blood cells and bacteria in the urine. Also, a sample of urine can be cultured in agar. There the microbes in the sample will grow and divide. Further tests can be performed to find out what microbes are present, and what antibiotic will kill them.

<u>Antibiotics</u>:
The drugs used are not the same as those used to treat Chlamydia or gonorrhea. The antibiotics used are those most active against microbes in the stool and skin. Treatment is prescribed for 3 to 10 days in simple cases.

<u>Partner notification</u>:
Cystitis is not spread by having sex. There is no need to inform or treat sexual partners.

CANDIDA (yeast) (also called "Monilia")
Vaginal yeast infection is very common. Some women have this many times or even all of the time. Women with diabetes get this often. Women who take antibiotics for any reason can get a yeast infection. The antibiotics kill "good" bacteria that are normally present in the vagina. This opens up a spot for the yeast to grow. The yeast causing this problem is called *Candida albicans*.

The most common symptom is an increased amount of vaginal discharge. This often contains whitish flecks. The skin in the region can become very red, tender, and itchy.

In normal cases there are no major complications.

T.A.P. for Candida (yeast)
<u>Tests</u>:
One can see the yeasts in the vaginal discharge under a microscope.
One can grow the yeasts in culture, but this is not done as a routine test.

<u>Antibiotics</u>:
Yeast infection needs to be treated only if it is causing symptoms.
Several drugs that kill yeasts (clotrimazole, miconazole, nystatin) can be
used. They are designed to be placed in the vagina in the form of a
suppository. They also can be applied as a lotion or cream. Treatment
often takes about 7 days.

<u>Partner notification</u>:
This is not required. Women who contract Candida get it for reasons that
have nothing to do with sex. In many persons yeast microbes are often
(always) present on the skin. Symptoms are caused by too much growth
of yeast in the vaginal area.

TRICHOMONAS
This microbe is a *protozoan* (a complex single-cell organism). It can
cause a burning feeling when passing urine. It also can cause an
increased vaginal discharge. This can be yellow or green in color and
frothy. With severe infection, vague pains can be felt in the lower
abdomen. The pains can be worse during sex.

Trichomonas can infect the cervix, also. Chronic infection with
trichomonas might lead to a slightly increased risk of cervical cancer.

T.A.P. for trichomonas

<u>Tests</u>:
Looking at the discharge under a microscope often will disclose the
microbes. They can be grown in culture, but this is not done as a routine
test.

<u>Antibiotics</u>:
The usual drugs are metronidazole or tinidazole. They can be given as one large single dose or in smaller amounts for up to 10 days. Patients should not drink alcohol while taking metronidazole. If they do, they will become very sick and nauseous. Metronidazole or tinidazole often are not given to women who are pregnant. These drugs pose a possible risk to the fetus. Vaginal suppositories containing other drugs are used.

<u>Partner notification</u>:
Trichomonas infection can be contracted by non-sexual means, but it also can be spread by having sex. Treatment of the sexual partner is needed to prevent re-infection.

A man infected with trichomonas may have a discharge and a burning sensation at the penis. More often, a "no symptom" infection will be present.

GARDNERELLA (bacterial vaginosis)
The cause is growth in the vagina of bacteria called *Gardnerella vaginalis*. Often other bacteria are found, also.

The usual symptom is a clear vaginal discharge which sometimes has a bad smell.

T.A.P. for Bacterial vaginosis (Gardnerella)
<u>Tests</u>:
Testing the vaginal discharge can point to this problem. If you add a chemical called potassium hydroxide, the discharge gives off a strange odor. The discharge is less acid than normal. This can be tested for using special paper. When you look at the discharge under a microscope, you can sometimes see cells coated with tiny Gardnerella bacteria.

<u>Antibiotics</u>:
This is treated with special antibiotics.

<u>Partner notification</u>:
Not required.

APPENDIX 2

Other causes of pimples, blisters, and sores

on the genitals

There are many causes other than syphilis, herpes-2, or genital warts (HPV). It is your doctor's job to find out what the cause is. This is not always easy.

COMMON CAUSES THAT ARE NOT STDs:
>   Acne pimples
>   Skin infection due to lack of cleanliness
>   Insect and spider bites
>   Heat rash
>   Candida (yeast)
>   Zipper cut
>   Other injury
>   Drug rash
>   Contact allergy
>   Psoriasis
>   Infected sebaceous cyst
>   Infected Bartholin's gland

Acne pimples are common in the genital region. They look like acne elsewhere in the body. Sometimes, though, herpes-2 can cause large "pimples" on the buttocks that look like acne.

Skin infection due to lack of cleanliness. Skin bacteria cause pimples and sores that can look like those caused by STD microbes.

An insect or spider bite can look like a syphilis sore.

Heat rash can cause pimples or sores in this region.

Candida (yeast): Yeast can cause the skin of the genital region to become red, tender, and itchy. The skin can break down to form a sore.

A **zipper cut** can get infected and turn into a sore that looks like a syphilis chancre. On the other hand, some persons who get a syphilis sore assume wrongly that it is a zipper cut. You get a sore on the penis that looks like a zipper cut. You don't recall hurting yourself in this way. You have been sexually active. What should you do? You need to get checked for syphilis.

Other injury: Injury during oral sex can cause a scrape or a sore on the penis or in vaginal area.

Drug rash: Patients who are allergic to a drug can break out in a rash. Sometimes the rash appears only in one part of the body. Such a rash is called a "fixed drug eruption". The penis is a common region for this to occur. The skin here can become red and swollen and may break open to form a sore.

Contact allergy: Sometimes an allergic reaction can happen in skin that has come into contact with an irritating substance. For instance, there may be an allergy to the latex rubber in condoms. In such a case, the skin of the penis can become red, swollen, and break open to form a sore.

Psoriasis: This is a skin disease that causes a scaly, crusty rash. Lesions can be present in the genital region and be confused with changes due to an STD.

Sebaceous glands are glands found under the skin. They produce an oily substance. If a gland gets blocked it can form a cyst. This can grow in size, get infected, and break open to form a sore.

Bartholin's glands are glands found at the vaginal inlet. They can become blocked and infected to form an abscess. Sometimes, infection

120

in these glands is due to gonorrhea microbes.

OTHER STDs THAT CAUSE PIMPLES OR SORES ON THE GENITALS
Scabies
Pubic lice
Molluscum contagiosum
Chancroid
Lymphogranuloma venereum
Granuloma inguinale

SCABIES (see APPENDIX 3)
Scabies can cause crusted sores.

CRAB LICE (see APPENDIX 4)
Crab lice can cause small blood-filled blisters.

MOLLUSCUM CONTAGIOSUM
This is an infection caused by a virus. It is spread by having sex, but it also can be spread by other close personal contact.

Molluscum contagiosum causes small, firm pimples in the genital region. The pimples may be the flesh-colored, white, yellow, or translucent. They can look pearly, smooth, and waxy. Often there is a tiny crater in the center. Most often the pimples do not cause pain. If untreated, some of them can turn into large sores.

T.A.P. for Molluscum Contagiosum
Tests
The pimples have a typical look to them. Scrapings from the opened pimple can be checked under the microscope. With molluscum contagiosum, one can see certain kinds of changes inside skin cells.

<u>Antibiotics</u>
There are no good drugs against this viral STD. Treatment is to destroy the lesions. The pimples are first opened. Then they are frozen by touching them with a probe cooled with liquid nitrogen. Another way is to burn them off chemically using silver nitrate or other compounds.

<u>Partner Notification</u>
The incubation period is thought to range from about 2 weeks to 6 months. Often a second STD will be found in sexual partners.

CHANCROID
Chancroid is caused by a bacterium. This STD causes sores that look like syphilis chancres. The sores appear 4-14 days after intimate sexual contact with an infected partner. About a week later, the lymph glands in the genital region become swollen.

The lymph glands can swell to a very large size. They can break down to form an abscess. Severe scarring can result. Sometimes lymph glands in the region of the rectum or vagina are involved. Then the tissue between the vagina and rectum can be destroyed. A hole can then open up between the rectum and vagina.

LYMPHOGRANULOMA VENEREUM (LGV)
This is a bacterial infection caused by a type of Chlamydia microbe. A sore may appear in the genital region 1 to 3 weeks after sex with an infected person. Several weeks later the local lymph glands become involved.

The complications of LGV are due to infection in the lymph glands. The lymph glands become swollen, form abscesses, and then form scar tissue. Sometimes the scar tissue becomes very thick. Then there can be chronic swelling of the genital organs or of the legs.

GRANULOMA INGUINALE

This STD is due to a bacterium, also. A sore appears on the genitals or around the anus 1-12 weeks after sex with an infected person. The sore can grow to be very large. Granuloma inguinale does not affect the lymph glands. Rarely, the infection can spread to other body organs such as the bones, joints, and liver.

T.A.P. for chancroid, LGV, and granuloma inguinale:
All are treated with antibiotics. Treatment must be given early, before scarring of lymph tissue occurs. For each of these infections, you should inform your present and recent sexual partners. Go back about 1-3 months from the time the first signs of infection appeared.

APPENDIX 3

Scabies

Scabies is an infection of the skin caused by a tiny insect or mite called *Sarcoptes scabiei*. Because scabies is spread by having sex, it is an STD. However, scabies also can be spread by close, non-sexual contact, and by way of shared bed linens and clothing.

The mites burrow into the skin to lay their eggs. A few weeks later the region begins to itch. Scratching causes crusty pimples to form.

Scabies can affect the skin of many parts of the body. The finger webs, forearms, and shins often are involved.

T.A.P. for Scabies:
Tests:
If you look under a microscope at a sample scraped from a scabies pimple, you might see one of the mites.

Antibiotics:
Drugs that kill scabies mites are sold in the form of a lotion. First, you shower and shampoo. Then you apply the lotion to the entire body (except the face) and rub it in gently. You wait 12 hours and then you wash the lotion off. You need to wash all of your bed linens and clothes to prevent re-infection.

Partner notification:
Yes. Also, all family members or persons sharing the household should be treated to prevent re-infection.

APPENDIX 4

Crab lice (Pediculosis)

Crab lice or "crabs" is caused by a louse, a small insect-like microbe that looks like a tiny crab under the microscope. The name of this louse is *Pthirus pubis*. The adult louse, about 1-2 mm in length, clings to pubic hairs close to the skin. It looks like a brown flake of dandruff. The louse lays its eggs, called *nits*, on the pubic hairs. The nits look like grains of rice. They hatch in 7-10 days.

Crabs or pubic lice are spread by having sex, so some consider this to be an STD. Even so, the lice also are spread by any type of close contact and even by sharing blankets or clothing. You can get crab lice from using a toilet seat that was used before you by a person with this infestation.

Crab lice feed on a person's blood. The feeding sites are marked by pinpoint red lesions. Crab lice can cause intense itching in the genital region. Scratching causes swollen, red, inflamed, and crusted skin lesions.

T.A.P. for pubic lice
Tests:
You might find a louse or its eggs attached to a pubic hair.

Antibiotics:
You use a lotion that contains a chemical that kills crab lice, such as pyrethin. You apply the lotion to the pubic region after bathing. Rinsing with vinegar can get the nits off of the pubic hairs.

Partner notification:
Yes. Also, all members of the household should be checked for crab lice and treated if need be. All clothing and bedding should be laundered.

APPENDIX 5

Viral Hepatitis

There are at least three types of hepatitis virus, types A, B, and C. The Greek word *hepar* means **liver**, and the word *hepatitis* means **inflammation of the liver**. These viruses all infect the liver. Type A hepatitis does not cause chronic (long-lasting) liver infection or damage. Types B and C virus do cause chronic infection. They can damage or scar the liver and cause other problems.

How hepatitis can be spread
Type A virus is present in the feces during infection. When persons with type A virus forget to wash their hands after touching their anal region, they can contaminate food with the virus. The virus can be spread to others when they ingest this food. This is called **fecal-oral** spread. Type A hepatitis can be spread by intimate sexual contact as well.

Types B and C hepatitis
These viruses are different from each other and from the type A virus. After they infect the liver, they can cause a chronic illness in the body. The B and C viruses can remain in the blood as well as in genital fluids for long periods of time.

Types B and C viruses can be spread by
- (1) intimate sexual contact
- (2) abuse of injectable drugs
- (3) contaminated blood products
- (4) other, non-sexual means

Blood from donors is now tested for hepatitis B and C. If the test is positive the blood is not used. These tests are not perfect.

Symptoms
Symptoms can appear from 2 weeks to 6 months after infection. They include:

> Fever
> Headache
> Poor appetite
> Nausea, vomiting
> Tiredness, weakness
> Jaundice (a yellow color of the skin or
> > of the "whites of the eyes")

Many persons with hepatitis have no symptoms!

T.A.P. for hepatitis
Tests:
Three types of blood tests are used. They measure blood levels of:
1) Liver enzymes
2) Antibodies to the virus
3) Viral DNA or other viral fragments

There can be a long "time-lag" between the moment you get hepatitis and the time that blood tests turn positive.

Antibiotics:
There are no good antiviral drugs for hepatitis. Usually no treatment is needed. There are some new drugs being tested to treat chronic hepatitis.

If you think you may have just been exposed to hepatitis, there is something you can do. You can get injections of antibodies (gamma globulin) obtained from the blood of healthy patients.

There is a very good vaccine against type B hepatitis. The vaccine must be given before exposure. Suppose you are sexually active and have many partners. Suppose you abuse injectable drugs. Then you are at risk for hepatitis B. You should get this vaccine.

Partner notification:
You are found to have hepatitis. You have had sex with others in the recent past. What should you do? Talk to your doctor or clinic for help about warning sexual partners. If you abused drugs and shared needles or other supplies with others, then those "partners" may need to be informed, also.

Glossary

abstinence--the holding back from, or staying away from something of one's own free will. For instance, you can decide to be abstinent from sex and drugs.

antibody--A protein made by the body that binds to a bacterium or virus and helps kill it.

antibiotic-- a drug that kills bacteria, fungus, virus, or other microbes.

bacteria--microbes composed of a single cell. Some bacteria such as Chlamydia, though, are not complete cells.

chancre--a sore caused by syphilis. It can appear on the genitals, the mouth, or on other parts of the body. A chancre contains many syphilis microbes.

chronic--long-lasting, drawn out.

condom--a thin sheath most often made of latex. A condom is shaped like a cylinder with one closed end. It is placed onto the penis before sex. A condom is designed to keep semen from the vagina. Use of a condom helps prevent the spread of STDs.

contagious--spread by direct or indirect contact.

culture--the growing of microbes on agar or in cells.

discharge--liquid composed of secretions and/or pus that flows from a body opening or wound.

fungus--a simple form of plant life made up of cells that do not contain chlorophyll. Some fungus can infect human tissues. The Candida microbe is a fungus (see also *yeast*).

genital--having to do with the sex organs.   In the male these include the penis, scrotum, and testicles. In the female, it refers mostly to the region of the vaginal opening and to the cervix.

groin--that part of the body where the thigh meets the trunk. The groin includes the genitals.

incubation period--the period from the time of entry of a microbe into the body to the first sign or symptom of disease.

infection--a condition that occurs when a microbe enters a part of the body and multiplies there to produce harmful effects. **Colonization**, on the other hand, is when microbes multiply in a part of the body but produce no harmful effects.

intravenous--within or into a vein.

"-itis"--when this ending is added to the name of a body part or organ, it means that the organ is infected. For instance, there is vaginitis (vagina), cystitis (bladder), cervicitis (cervix), salpingitis (salpinges, or Fallopian tubes), urethritis (urethra), proctitis (proctum=another word for rectum).

lymph vessels and glands--the lymph vessels form a network of tissue spaces and tubes. The lymph vessels work like storm sewers. They pick up any excess fluid or protein that has seeped into tissue spaces and route it back to the blood. Every so often, the lymph vessels enter small, rounded, **lymph nodes** or **glands**. In lymph nodes there are large numbers of white blood cells. They stop and kill any microbes that have entered the lymph fluid. During infection, the lymph nodes can swell and become painful.

masturbation--when one strokes or rubs (with the fingers) the penis or vaginal region with the purpose of getting sexually aroused, often to the point orgasm.

culture medium--a broth that contains minerals and nutrients. It can be made solid by adding a gel-like substance called agar. Culture medium is used to grow microbes so that they can be identified.

microbe--a very small life form, usually a bacteria, fungus, yeast, or virus.

monogamy--the state of being married to or having sex with only one person.

nonoxynol-9--a chemical that kills sperm. It can kill some STD microbes, also, when used with a condom.

134

Pap test--a test named after its inventor, Dr. Papanicolaou. The test is to look under a microscope at cells scraped from the cervix to check for cancer.

protein--a molecule containing nitrogen, carbon, hydrogen, oxygen, and occasionally, other elements. Proteins are one of the building blocks for human tissues.

pustule--a pimple filled with fluid. The fluid inside often contains microbes and white blood cells.

reagin--an antibody made by white blood cells that appears in the blood in patients with syphilis

recurrence--return of symptoms after a period of no symptoms.

rectum--that lowermost part of the large intestine that opens into the anus.

risk--possible or probable danger or harm.

screening test--a quick, simple test that suggests (but doesn't always prove) that a given disease may be present.

secretion--liquid produced by cells lining the opening of an organ or gland. A secretion can flow into a body cavity (saliva, vaginal secretions) or into the blood.

symptom--a change in the body or its functions that can be noticed and that may be due to disease.

venereal disease--an old term for STD (sexually transmitted disease). The word "venereal" comes from the name "Venus", the ancient Roman goddess of love.

yeast--a very small fungus (see above) that divides by budding. The Candida microbe is a fungus, and it also is a yeast.

REVIEW QUESTIONS

WHAT IS AN STD?

1. Colds and some diarrheal infections are caused by viruses or bacteria. Colds and infectious diarrhea can be spread by playing with an infected person, by kissing, or by eating at the same table. Why is it that STDs are not spread in this manner? STDs are caused by viruses or bacteria, also.

There are a few key differences between the microbes that cause colds and diarrhea and the microbes that cause STD. The colds and diarrhea microbes can survive for some time outside of the body. Colds viruses are present in sputum and in mucus in the nose. When someone sneezes or coughs, these viruses are spread into the air or onto objects. They can be inhaled by other people, or picked up by the hands and transferred into the mouth. In infectious diarrhea, the microbes are present in the feces. If an infected person doesn't wash his or her hands after wiping, the virus can be transferred to foods or other objects, and then enter another person's body through the mouth.

STD viruses and bacteria are not present in sputum, nasal mucus, or feces, in amounts high enough to transmit infection. Also, STD viruses and bacteria are not very hardy, and don't usually survive for long periods of time outside of the body.

STD viruses and bacteria are present in secretions and pus coming from infected sex organs. STDs are spread when these infected secretions come into direct contact with a body orifice of a second person during sex.

Because HIV (the virus that causes AIDS) can be present in the blood of infected persons, HIV can be spread by use of contaminated needles, syringes, or injectable drugs.

2. Circle the risk behaviors that often result in spread of an STD:
a) Hugging
b) Deep kissing or fondling another person's sex organs with the hands
c) Intimate sex involving contact between the penis and vagina or anus
d) Intimate sex involving contact between the mouth and penis
e) Living in the same family with an infected person
f) Eating at the same table with an infected person
g) Kissing a person who has a herpes or syphilis sore on the lips.
h) Swimming in a pool used by an infected person.
i) Injecting yourself with drugs (when not being supervised by a doctor).
Answer: c,d,g,i;   Comments: (b) is possible but very unlikely

3. What about wrestling and sports where people get bloody noses and cuts? Is there a danger of getting HIV/AIDS by taking part in such sports?
Herpes (mostly type 1) can be spread during wrestling. At time of this writing (1992), there is no evidence that HIV/AIDS or any of the other major STDs can be spread by taking part in sports. You should always try to avoid contact with another person's blood during sports. If blood is spilled on the floor, the area should be cleaned up wearing gloves. The area should be cleaned with a mixture of 1 part bleach and 9 parts water. Bloody towels should be washed using detergent and hot water.

4. John told Mary, "I've had a vasectomy. Don't worry about getting an STD from me." Right or wrong?
Wrong. A vasectomy is when a surgeon cuts the tube connecting the testicles (where sperm are made) and the urethra. If John has an STD, then gonorrhea or Chlamydia microbes can be present in his urethra. If John has syphilis, herpes-2, or genital warts, the microbes might be present in sores or warts on the skin. Mary can get an STD from a man who's had a vasectomy!

5. Why is the rate of STDs so high?
Many persons continue to engage in unsafe sex with many partners. Injecting oneself with drugs using contaminated needles also is a factor.

6. How are Chlamydia, gonorrhea, and syphilis alike?
All are caused by bacteria.

7. How are herpes-2, genital warts (HPV), and HIV alike?
All are caused by viruses.

138

SYMPTOMS

1. Which STDs can be present without causing symptoms?
All of the ones discussed: Chlamydia, gonorrhea, syphilis, herpes-2, genital warts (HPV), and HIV.

2. How are Chlamydia and gonorrhea alike?
Both cause the same type of symptoms (discharge and/or burning). Both can infect the Fallopian tubes. Both can scar and block these tubes. Then the woman can't get pregnant. She may have an ectopic pregnancy, causing severe bleeding.

3. How are the symptoms of syphilis and herpes-2 alike?
Both cause sores on the sex organs.

4. How are symptoms of syphilis and herpes-2 different?
The syphilis chancre is usually a single lesion that is painless. Herpes-2 sores are multiple, and they start off as blisters. Herpes-2 sores usually are painful. Syphilis can cause late (after many years) damage to brain, spinal cord, and heart.

5. Which STDs are associated with an increased risk of cancer of the cervix?
Herpes-2, genital warts, and maybe, trichomonas (see Appendix 1).

6. What's the difference between a cold sore and a herpes-2 sore?
Cold sores are caused by a related virus, herpes-1. Herpes-1 also can cause sores on the genitals. Most people have been infected with herpes-1 at one time or another. Many are partially immune.

7. If you have a cold sore on the lips, should you be careful not to kiss anyone?
This depends on who the person is. Kissing another adult may be OK, as most adults have been infected by herpes-1 already. However, some adults who have never been exposed to herpes-1 may get very severe disease. You should never kiss a baby or child while you have the sore. Babies probably will not have had herpes-1. They could get a severe case of herpes-1 in this way.

8. What is the difference between HIV and AIDS?
HIV means that the virus is inside the body, multiplying in white blood cells and other tissues. HIV causes damage to white blood cells, leading to **A**cquired **I**mmuno**D**eficiency **S**yndrome or AIDS. Immunodeficiency means the inability to fight infection. This can lead to severe pneumonia, growth of tumors (Kaposi's sarcoma), and death.

9. Which STDs are often fatal (cause death)?
HIV is the only STD that is often fatal.

10. What are the two risk behaviors that can result in getting HIV?
Sex with an infected person, and injecting drugs using needles or other material that has become contaminated with HIV from being used beforehand by an infected person. HIV also can be spread from mother to child. It can be spread by transfusion of infected blood products. Transfusion now has a very low risk, since all donated blood is screened for HIV before use (the test isn't perfect).

11. What are the symptoms of HIV?
Usually none. Some persons get a flu-like illness a few weeks or months after infection. Symptoms of AIDS (Acquired Immunodeficiency Syndrome) may not appear for 10 years or more. AIDS symptoms are listed in the answer to #13.

12. Can Chlamydia, gonorrhea, syphilis, herpes-2, or genital warts be transmitted by injecting illegal drugs? Why yes or why no?
Syphilis microbes can be found in the blood of infected persons, but we don't know for sure if syphilis can be spread in this way. The other microbes usually are not present in the blood and are not spread by contaminated needles.

13. What are the symptoms of AIDS?
Fatigue, weight loss, and diarrhea. There is low resistance to infection. Severe pneumonia can result. There may be confusion and poor memory if the brain is affected. Tumors called Kaposi's sarcoma may cause bluish marks on the skin.

14. I am in a relationship where I am having sex. Lately I've noticed a discharge and burning feeling at the tip of my penis. Do I have an STD?
Probably. If the discharge occurs throughout the day and if there is burning when passing urine, the chances are good you have an STD. You need to be checked for gonorrhea and Chlamydia.

15. *I've noticed a large amount of vaginal discharge. The vaginal region is very red, tender, and itchy. I haven't had sex in the past 6 months. Do I have an STD?*
Probably not. There are many conditions that are not STDs that cause these symptoms, such as yeast. Also, you may have an infection of the urine due to bacteria coming from the stool or skin (see Appendix 1).

16. *Besides syphilis, herpes-2, and genital warts, what other conditions can cause sores on the sex organs?*
There are many non-STD causes, such as acne, skin infection due to poor hygiene, and insect bites. Also, other STDs can cause such sores. See Appendix 2.

DURING PREGNANCY

1. *Of the six STDs discussed, which can be spread to the baby during birth?*
Chlamydia, gonorrhea, syphilis, herpes-2, and HIV. Spread of genital warts (HPV) from mother to baby can also occur, but this is uncommon.

2. *Which STDs cause an eye infection in the newborn.?*
Chlamydia and gonorrhea.

3. *Which STDs can infect the fetus while it is still in the womb?*
Syphilis. HIV also might be spread at this stage.

4. *Which STDs are very serious in the newborn?*
Herpes-2 (neurologic disease) and syphilis (damage to many organ systems). HIV also is very serious (it often leads to death), but usually HIV doesn't cause symptoms until several months to years after birth.

5. *Is it possible to prevent spread of STDs to the fetus or newborn?*
Yes, partially. In the case of syphilis, by early treatment of the mother with antibiotics. The risk of eye infection by gonorrhea or Chlamydia can be reduced by putting antibiotic drops into the baby's eyes after birth. The risk of herpes-2 can be reduced by taking the baby out through the abdomen by surgery (Caesarean section).

LABORATORY TESTS

1. My doctor took a sample of my discharge and put it in a dish full of nutrient to see if any STD microbes would grow. What STDs was he checking for?
Gonorrhea. Chlamydia microbes also can be grown in culture, but they grow only in cells. The usual test for Chlamydia is to mix the discharge with antibodies that have been tagged with a dye or enzyme.

2. Which STDs are checked for by a blood test?
Syphilis and HIV.

3. Which STDs are checked for by looking at scrapings from sores under a microscope?
Syphilis and herpes-2.

4. What is the time lag effect? Why is it important?
Blood tests for syphilis and HIV may not turn positive until up to 3 months (syphilis) or 6 months (HIV) after infection. If you think you may have gotten syphilis or HIV, a negative blood test taken soon afterwards doesn't mean that you are in the clear. You need to take a repeat blood test in 3 months (syphilis) or in 3-6 months (HIV).

5. I think I might have HIV. I am thinking of having the blood test. What are the good points and bad points of being tested?
Bad points: If you find out you have HIV, this may be tough for you to bear. You might get depressed. If you tell the wrong person about your test results, word might leak out that you have HIV. You might then lose some friends. It might be hard for you to get a job, even though in many regions there are laws that say you can't discriminate against persons with HIV. You may not be able to get life insurance.
Reasons to take the HIV blood test: HIV can be fatal. If you have HIV, you need to know. Taking some of the newer drugs might delay the onset of AIDS. If you know you have HIV, then you need to abstain from sex. If you know which person you got HIV from, these people need to know, also. This is the only way that we can stop the spread of HIV. HIV testing is almost always done in a way that keeps the results secret from people who have no business knowing the results. Your friends or your coworkers will not know the results of your test unless you tell them. In almost all cases, if you think you may have gotten HIV through sex or through injecting drugs, the right decision is to be tested for HIV. You should have one test now and a second test 3-6 months later. Most clinics offer counseling to people who are thinking about taking the test.

142

TREATMENT

1. What is the T.A.P. system for treating STDs?
The letters stand for **T**ests, **A**ntibiotics, and **P**artner notification.

2. Some STDs are caused by bacteria; others are caused by viruses. How does this affect their treatment?
Chlamydia, gonorrhea, and syphilis are caused by bacteria. Each can be cured with antibiotics if treated early. Herpes-2, genital warts, and HIV all are due to viruses. They cannot be fully cured at this time. Genital warts can be removed, and often don't come back, though. Drugs against viruses are new and need more work. Some antiviral drugs can partly block the symptoms of herpes-2, and they can lower the rate at which herpes-2 sores keep coming back. Other antiviral drugs may delay the weakening of the immune system due to HIV. There are drugs that help prevent *Pneumocystis carinii* pneumonia in patients with AIDS.

3. Can one antibiotic cure both Chlamydia and gonorrhea?
Not usually. Because many persons are infected with both types of microbes, two different drugs often are given. Some new drugs, though, may be active against both microbes at the same time.

4. If I have an STD, will it go away if I take penicillin without going to a doctor?
Probably not. Gonorrhea microbes often are resistant to penicillin. Chlamydia microbes usually aren't affected by penicillin. To cure syphilis, penicillin must be given for a prolonged period of time, or a long-lasting type of shot needs to be given. Penicillin will have no effect on STDs due to viruses (herpes-2, genital warts, HIV).

5. What type of doctors treat STDs?
Any type. Your family practitioner or your pediatrician. Gynecologists often treat STDs in women. Urologists treat men with STDs. Dermatologists are consulted to find the cause of sores or rashes. Public Health Clinics or STD clinics run by University or Hospital Medical Centers are other good places to go.

6. I got an STD from my sex partner. He/she gave me this infection. Why should I bother to tell him/her?
STDs often cause no symptoms. Your partner may not know that he/she has an STD. STDs can be dangerous. Morally, it is your duty to warn someone of a danger of which they may not be aware. Also, your partner may have had sex with other

persons and infected them also. These other people may need to be warned. This is best done with the help of your public health clinic.

7. Are there any legal problems about warning partners about an STD?
Persons have been sued for knowingly spreading an STD. In some regions it is a crime to knowingly spread an STD to others.

8. I just got symptoms of Chlamydia/gonorrhea/herpes-2 for the first time yesterday. Is there any point to my notifying a person that I had sex with 2 months ago?
Ask your doctor. Each case is different. Having said this, symptoms of these three STDs usually appear within one month of having sex. The person you had sex with 2 months ago probably is not the cause of your STD.

9. What about genital warts, syphilis, or HIV?
These infections have much longer "incubation periods". Someone you had sex with 2 months ago (or even longer) might have become infected from you or might have given you the STD. This person should be informed.

PREVENTION

1. How do I avoid getting an STD?
Postpone sex until marriage (or the same type of stable, adult relationship). Don't inject yourself with illegal drugs or steroids. Don't get a tattoo or get involved with needle-sticks from blood-brother pacts, etc. If you are having sex, don't have sex with strangers or with many partners. Always use a latex condom. Use nonoxynol-9 along with the condom.

2. How effective are latex condoms in preventing STDs?
If you use condoms the right way and always, they can give you good protection against getting Chlamydia, gonorrhea, and HIV. However, the protection is far from perfect. AIDS is a fatal disease. If you know that a person has HIV, you shouldn't have sex with him/her, even when using a condom. Use of a latex condom will protect you to some extent against syphilis, herpes-2, or genital warts. However, these microbes are very contagious. They may be present in sores or warts located outside of the region covered by a condom.

144

3. *Will taking antibiotics before sex stop me from getting an STD? Will washing after sex keep me from getting an STD?*
No and no.

4. *What are key actions of a good decision maker?*
You think in advance about each course of action. Then you compare the possible consequences of each alternative.

5. *How do you say "NO" effectively if you really don't want to do something?*
See pages 99-100.

CASE HISTORIES

1. *What is one point made by the story "SPRING BREAK"?*
Don't have sex with strangers.

2. *What is one point made by the story "PARTY"?*
Bad situations can get you into trouble. When you see that things are getting out of control, remove yourself as soon as you can.

3. *What lessons can be drawn from "MACHO MAN?".*
   a) Persons who have sex with many partners have a higher than normal risk of having an STD.
   b) Henry didn't know how to use a condom because he never had any training. Suppose he had taken a good sex education program. There he might have learned how to use a condom in the right way.
   c) Persons who have many sex partners often find it hard to relate to any one person for a long period. Suppose you get involved with someone like this. You may find that he/she does not want a lasting relationship.

4. *What lessons can be drawn from "TIME BOMB?".*
After getting HIV, you (or your partner) can feel fine for many years. Symptoms may take 10 years or more to show up.

AIDS AND STD TELEPHONE HOTLINES:

UNITED STATES OF AMERICA
National HIV and AIDS Information Service:

    1-800-342-AIDS (24 hours a day, 7 days/week)

    1-800-344-SIDA (in Spanish, 8:00 AM to 2:00 AM, 7 days/week)

    1-800-243-7889 (TTY/TDD line for the hearing impaired)

The National STD Hotline

    1-800-227-8922 (Mon-Fri, 8:00 A.M. to 11:00 P.M. EST)

    1-809-765-1010 (in Spanish in Puerto Rico; NOT a toll-free call,

                           but collect calls accepted. Mon-Fri, 7:00 AM-10:30 PM)

CANADA

Federal Center for AIDS	613-725-3769
Canadian AIDS Society	613-230-3580
National AIDS Clearinghouse	613-725-3769
Alberta	800-722-AIDS
British Columbia	800-972-2437
Manitoba	800-782-AIDS
New Brunswick	506-459-7518
Newfoundland	709-576-3430
North West Territories	800-661-0795
Nova Scotia	902-424-8698
Ontario	800-267-7432 (English)
	800-668-2437 (French)
Prince Edward Island	902-368-4965
Quebec	800-463-5656
Saskatchewan	306-787-3148
Yukon	403-668-6461

UNITED KINGDOM

National AIDS Helpline

    0800 567123 24 hours a day. Free

    0800 521361 Minicom for the hearing impaired

                10 A.M.-10 P.M. daily

    0800 282445 Bengali, Gujarati, Hindi, Punjabi, Urdu;

    0800 282446 Cantonese 6-10 P.M. Tuesdays

    0800 282447 Arabic 6-10 P.M. Wednesdays

UNITED KINGDOM (continued)

Scottish AIDS Monitor	031 557 3885	
Northern Irish AIDS Helpline	0232 326117	7:30-10 P.M. MWF
Cardiff AIDS Helpline	0222 223443	7-10 P.M. weekdays
Mainliners	071 737 3141	For those affected by HIV and drugs
Body Positive	071 373 9124	Calls are taken by people who are HIV+.

Terrence Higgins Trust

Helpline	071 242 1010	3-10 P.M. Daily
Legal Line	071 405 2381	7-10 P.M. Wednesdays

IRELAND
Cork AIDS Helpline	276 676
Dublin AIDS Helpline	724 277

NEW ZEALAND
AIDS Helpline	395 560	National Toll-Free Number

AUSTRALIA
South Australia AIDS Line	008 888 559	
	083 621 611	
Queensland AIDS Council	884 1990	24 hours
	008 177 434	9 A.M. - 5 P.M. Free.
Tasmania AIDS line	002 311 930	
Victoria AIDS line	034 836 700	
	008 134 840	7-10 P.M. Free.
Western Australia AIDS line	092 278 355	9 A.M. - 10 P.M.
	008 199 287	9 A.M. - 5 P.M. Free.
AIDS Council New South Wales	022 833 222	Mon-Fri 10 A.M. - 5 P.M.
Sydney AIDS Hotline	332 4000	10 A.M. - 10 P.M.
AIDS Action Council of ACT	062 572 855	
AIDS Council of Central Australia	089 531 118	
Northern Territories AIDS Line	089 411 711	

How to order copies of this book:

Institutions must send a purchase order number.
Individuals must prepay by check.

Individual copy price: $14.95
Shipping (within the USA/CANADA): $1.50 for first book
                                     $0.50 for each additional book
International shipping and tariffs billed separately.

Discounts: Very substantial discounts (>50%) available for classroom sets and other large orders.

Send orders to:
        Medtext, Inc.
        15W560 89th St.
        Hinsdale, IL 60521 USA
        (708)-325-3277

Note to health educators:
This book has been continually improved in response to your valuable suggestions. Your input and suggestions for change are very desirable and will be reflected in future editions. Please address all comments to the Editorial Office, Medtext, Inc., at the above address.